Contemporary Guide to Dermatology™

John Koo, MD
Director
Psoriasis Treatment Center
University of California Medical Center,
San Francisco

Lawrence C.C. Cheung, MD
Assistant Clinical Professor
Department of Dermatology
University of California, San Francisco

Chai Sue Lee, MD
Assistant Professor
Department of Dermatology
University of California, Davis

First Edition

D0814555

Published by Handbooks in Health Care Co.,
Newtown, Pennsylvania, USA

International Standard Book Number: 978-1-931981-74-3

Library of Congress Catalog Card Number: 2006940886

Web site: www.HHCbooks.com

Table of Contents

This book has been prepared and is presented as a service to the medical community. The information provided reflects the knowledge, experience, and personal opinions of the authors, John Koo, MD, Director, Psoriasis Treatment Center, University of California Medical Center, San Francisco; Lawrence C. C. Cheung, MD, Assistant Clinical Professor, Department of Dermatology, University of California, San Francisco; and Chai Sue Lee, MD, Assistant Professor, Department of Dermatology, University of California, Davis.

This book is not intended to replace or to be used as a substitute for the complete prescribing information prepared by each manufacturer for each drug. Because of possible variations in drug indications, in dosage information, in newly described toxicities, in drug/drug interactions, and in other items of importance, reference to such complete prescribing information is definitely recommended before any of the drugs discussed are used or prescribed.

Foreword

T he field of dermatology is ever-growing and offers clinicians many challenges, especially in reaching an accurate diagnosis and in selecting effective treatment options. Accurate diagnosis is particularly important at a time when patients are demanding prompt resolution of discomforting or disfiguring skin lesions. Unfortunately, in most medical schools, dermatologic disorders receive minimal attention, even though some of these disorders are increasing in incidence and in treatment resistance. Medical students, residents, and neophyte dermatologists have a multitude of options in learning about treatment choices. That is why this clinical handbook, *Contemporary Guide to Dermatology*™, is so useful. It offers practical information in a concise, readable manner, and uses evidence-based charts and tables to clarify pharmacologic options.

Drs. Koo, Cheung, and Lee explain the classifications of lesions as well as the diagnostic techniques of disorders by region of the most common dermatologic diseases. But the heart of the handbook is the authors' well-written examination of the most common individual disease states and the treatment options available.

For each disease state—such as acne vulgaris or dermatitis or psoriasis—the authors provide an overview, followed by a clinical description with points aimed at differential diagnosis, and then list the various approved treatment modalities. One of the most useful features of the handbook is the inclusion of the trade as well as generic names of all drugs. As all practicing physicians (including dermatologists) know, the number of available dermatologic drugs and their many formulations (eg, oral and intravenous agents, topical gels and creams, dermatologic washes) are staggering.

The handbook also emphasizes the potential side effects of dermatologic agents, a critical consideration in patient compliance and treatment efficacy. Another convenient feature of the handbook is the insert of full-color clinical photographs that depict a variety of skin disorders.

Finally, the handbook steadfastly focuses on relevant clinical information organized and formatted for quick reference and leaves the more esoteric topics for the much bigger textbooks. In doing so, the authors have put together a practice-based and easy-to-read authoritative handbook that clinicians can use with confidence.

Madhavi Kandula, MD
Clinical Instructor
Washington University School of Medicine
St. Louis, Missouri
and Dermatologist in private practice

Chapter **1**

Dermatologic Diagnosis and Classification

S kin diseases are common. Approximately 7% of yearly outpatient visits in the United States are for dermatologic complaints. The incidence is likely to be higher in a pediatric practice. Only one third of these patients are seen by dermatologists; most are seen by primary care physicians.

Although thousands of skin disorders have been described, only a small number account for most patient visits. The purpose of this handbook is to familiarize the reader with these common skin diseases.

Classification of Lesions

Lesions are classified into 13 categories, as listed in Table 1-1.

Classification of Surface Changes

Surface changes are classified into seven categories, as listed in Table 1-2.

Regional Diagnoses of Skin Disorders

Many skin conditions have a predilection for certain areas of the body, which may be helpful diagnostically. Table 1-3 lists common growths and rashes encountered in each region, listed in decreasing order of frequency.

Table 1-1: Classifications of Dermatologic Lesions

Lesion	Definition
Macule	flat circumscribed discoloration of skin, <1 cm in diameter
Patch	flat circumscribed discoloration of skin, >1 cm in diameter
Papule	discrete raised lesion, <1 cm in diameter
Plaque	discrete raised lesion, >1 cm in diameter
Vesicle	fluid-filled blister, <5 mm in diameter
Bulla	fluid-filled blister, >5 mm in diameter
Pustule	pus-filled blister
Fissure	crack in the epidermis
Erosion	partial loss of epidermis
Ulcer	complete loss of epidermis
Wheal	transient erythematous papule/plaque, generally describes urticarial lesions
Petechia	purple discoloration of the skin caused by extravasation of blood, <5 mm in diameter
Purpura	purple discoloration of the skin caused by extravasation of blood, >5 mm in diameter

Diagnostic Procedures

Skin Biopsy

A skin biopsy should be considered when lesions are suspected of neoplasia; for bullous disorders; ulcers not related to vascular insufficiency; and if the diagnosis remains uncertain after clinical examination.

For site selection, choose well-developed lesions; consider multiple biopsies of varying stages; and choose

Table 1-2: Classification of Dermatologic Surface Changes

- *Scaling* is flakes of loose cells derived from the stratum corneum (top epidermal layer).
- *Oozing* is seeping of fluid onto the surface of the lesions.
- *Crusting* is dried remains of serum (usually yellow).
- *Excoriation* refers to a lesion that has been scratched.
- *Lichenification* is thickening of the epidermis with exaggeration of skin lines.
- *Atrophy* is loss of thickness of the epidermis.
- *Lipoatrophy* is loss of subcutaneous fat.

vesicles, bullae, and pustules that are <24 to 48 hours old. When choosing the expanding border of large lesions also include a margin of normal skin for comparison.

For punch biopsy, subcutaneous fat should be included when possible, avoiding lesions with secondary changes (ie, infection and excoriation). Avoid knees, elbows, palms, and soles if possible; and avoid areas at risk for poor circulation or poor healing (ie, shin area on an elderly diabetic patient).

If a bleeding disorder is suspected, check CBC (complete blood count), PT/PTT (prothrombin time/partial thromboplastin time), and bleeding time. If platelets are >10,000/mm^3, a small punch biopsy is fine. When platelets are <10,000/mm^3, a punch biopsy should be delayed.

Aspirin should be held 9 to 10 days before biopsy, if possible, and can be resumed 1 day after the biopsy.

For small biopsies, warfarin (Coumadin®) may be continued during the biopsy. Otherwise, with low-risk conditions (deep vein thrombosis, stroke prevention, atrial

Table 1-3: Regional Diagnoses of Common Skin Disorders

Growths	Rashes
Scalp	
• Nevus	• Seborrheic dermatitis (dandruff)
• Seborrheic keratosis	• Psoriasis
• Pilar cyst	
• Actinic keratosis	
Face	
• Nevus	• Acne
• Lentigo	• Seborrheic dermatitis
• Actinic keratosis	• Rosacea
• Seborrheic keratosis (cosmetics)	• Contact dermatitis
• Sebaceous hyperplasia	• Herpes simplex
• Basal cell carcinoma	• Impetigo
• Squamous cell carcinoma	• Atopic dermatitis
• Flat wart	
Trunk	
• Nevus	• Acne
• Skin tag	• Tinea versicolor
• Cherry hemangioma	• Psoriasis
• Seborrheic keratosis	• Pityriasis rosea
• Epidermal inclusion cyst	• Scabies
• Lipoma	• Drug eruption
• Basal cell carcinoma	• Varicella
• Keloid	
• Neurofibroma	

Growths	Rashes
Genitalia	
• Wart (condyloma acuminatum)	• Herpes simplex
	• Scabies
• Molluscum contagiosum chronicus	• Psoriasis
	• Lichen simplex
Groin (Inguinal)	
• Skin tag	• Intertrigo
• Wart	• Tinea cruris
• Molluscum contagiosum	• Candidiasis
• Psoriasis	
• Pediculosis pubis	
Extremities	
• Nevus	• Atopic dermatitis
• Wart	• Contact dermatitis (from plants)
• Dermatofibroma	
• Seborrheic keratosis	• Psoriasis
• Actinic keratosis	• Insect bites
	• Drug eruption
	• Lichen planus (wrists and ankles)
	• Stasis dermatitis (legs)
	• Vasculitis (legs)
Hands (Dorsa)	
• Wart	• Contact dermatitis (occupational)
• Actinic keratosis	
• Actinic lentigo	• Scabies (interdigital)
• Squamous cell carcinoma	

(continued on next page)

Table 1-3: Regional Diagnoses of Common Skin Disorders
(continued)

Growths	Rashes
Hands (Palmar)	
• Wart	• Nonspecific eczematous dermatitis
	• Atopic dermatitis
	• Psoriasis
	• Tinea manuum
Feet (Dorsal)	
• Wart (shoe)	• Contact dermatitis
Feet (Plantar)	
• Wart (plantar)	• Tinea pedis
• Corn	• Nonspecific eczematous dermatitis
• Nevus	• Psoriasis
	• Atopic dermatitis

Adapted from Lookingbill DP, Marks JG Jr: *Principles of Dermatology*. Philadelphia, PA, WB Saunders Co, 1986.

fibrillation, status postmyocardial infarction, and/or stroke), hold 3 days before biopsy and resume 1 day after biopsy without loading dose. With high-risk conditions (hypercoagulable state and prosthetic valves), hold warfarin 1 week before biopsy. Continue subcutaneous heparin 500 mg b.i.d. through biopsy, and resume medication after the biopsy.

Fixatives: Formalin is adjusted 10% with phosphate buffer to pH 7.0. During the winter months, switch to

Table 1-4: Commonly Used Anesthetic Agents and Duration of Action

Agent	Duration of Action
Mepivacaine (Carbocaine®)	90 min
Lidocaine/epinephrine	180 min
Mepivacaine/epinephrine	180 min
Bupivacaine (Marcaine®)/epinephrine	200 min

the following to avoid freezing during transport: 70% ethanol and AAF (acetic acid/alcohol/formalin). Enzyme istochemistry/immunohistochemistry requires a special transport medium.

Anesthesia: Commonly used anesthetic agents are listed in Table 1-4. Epinephrine is contraindicated in end-vasculature areas (ie, digits, ears). Use a 3-mL to 10-mL syringe attached to a 30-gauge needle, 0.5 inches long. Mark the area to be biopsied because an introduction of anesthetic may distort landmarks. Inject into the center of the lesion, and do not inject directly into cystic lesions but around them (ring block). Inject anesthetic slowly, since this is the most painful part. If multiple injections are required, inject into previously anesthetized areas.

Punch Biopsy

The punch biopsy is a quick, simple procedure that produces a specimen core consisting of the epidermis, dermis, and part of the subcutaneous tissue (Table 1-5). The punch biopsy instrument is a disposable tubular knife analogous to a cookie cutter. Although the diameter of the punch biopsy knife usually ranges from 2 mm to 6 mm, the most popular sizes are 3 mm and 4 mm because smaller sizes may be

Table 1-5: Instructions for Punch Biopsy

1. Clean biopsy site, leaving scales and vesicles intact.

2. Consider marking the site before administration of anesthesia because local anesthetic may distort the anatomy.

3. Inject anesthesia into the center of the lesion at the dermal level to produce a wheal.

4. Use a rotational motion of the punch biopsy knife to produce the incision.

5. Be sure that the knife goes through the subcutaneous layer.

6. Exert downward pressure around the incision to force the biopsy specimen to elevate.

7. Be gentle if picking up the specimen with a pair of forceps, so as to not crush the specimen.

8. If necessary, use the anesthesia syringe needle to 'spear' the specimen at the level of the subcutaneous tissue to avoid crushing the specimen.

9. Use shears to transect the specimen at the level of the subcutaneous tissue.

10. Close the biopsy site, usually by sutures or by filling it with oxidized cellulose.

inadequate to interpret inflammatory processes. Choosing the correct site to biopsy based on the previously outlined criteria is paramount.

Clean the biopsy site, leaving scales and vesicles intact and consider marking the site before anesthesia because local anesthetic may distort the anatomy. Anesthetic is injected into the lesion's center at the dermal level to produce a wheal. Rotate the punch biopsy knife to produce the inci-

Table 1-6: Instructions for Shave Biopsy

1. Clean the biopsy site.

2. Inject anesthesia into the lesion at the dermal level to produce a wheal, elevating it from the surrounding normal tissue.

3. With the scalpel blade, cut under the lesion at the base of the elevated wheal in a horizontal plane parallel to the skin surface.

4. Achieve hemostasis with aluminum chloride. Avoid silver nitrate because it may leave a permanent stain on the skin.

5. Leave the deep dermis intact, and the area will heal without the need for sutures.

6. Instruct the patient about follow-up care.

sion. Be sure the knife goes through into the subcutaneous layer. Downward pressure around the incision will force the biopsy specimen to elevate and, if picking up the specimen with a pair of forceps, be gentle to avoid crushing it. The anesthesia syringe needle can be used to 'spear' the specimen at the level of the subcutaneous tissue to avoid crushing it. Shears are used to transect the specimen at the level of the subcutaneous tissue. The biopsy site is usually closed by sutures or filled in with oxidized cellulose.

Shave Biopsy

In this procedure, the shaving incision should be made at the level of the midreticular dermis, leaving the deep dermis intact and producing specimen that consists of the epidermis and the papillary dermis (Table 1-6). Therefore, this procedure should be reserved only for superficial processes (ie, nodular basal cell carcinoma, squamous cell carcinoma). Shave biopsy is not recommended if melanoma is suspected, since the accurate determination of the depth of the melanoma is critical in assessing prognosis.

Clean the biopsy site and then inject the lesion with anesthetic at the dermal level to produce a wheal, which elevates it from the surrounding normal tissue. Use a scalpel blade to cut under the lesion at the base of the elevated wheal in a horizontal plane parallel to the skin surface. Hemostasis is then achieved with aluminum chloride. Silver nitrate is best avoided since it may leave a permanent stain on the skin. If the deep dermis is left intact, the area will heal without sutures. The patient will then need instruction regarding follow-up care.

Potassium Hydroxide Mount

Potassium hydroxide (KOH) mounts identify the presence of fungal or yeast infections. Fungal cultures should be obtained if the species needs to be identified.

Skin: Scrapings should be taken from the active border of the lesion. Use a glass slide or a #15 scalpel to gently scrape the specimen onto another glass slide, and move the scrapings into the center of the slide with either another glass slide or a coverslip. Cover the slide with a coverslip and add several drops of KOH 10% to 30% solution at the edge of the coverslip. The KOH solution will be drawn under the coverslip via capillary action, eliminating air bubbles. Gently heat the slide, preferably with an alcohol lamp or by other means, which does not leave too much soot under the glass slide (be sure to avoid boiling the content). Allow the specimen to stand for a few minutes before examining it under a microscope. The specimen should be examined for hyphae, spores, and budding cells.

Hair: Specimens should be several freshly epilated hairs, which are placed on a slide with a coverslip. Add several drops of KOH 10% to 30% solution at the edge of the coverslip, and the KOH solution will be drawn under the coverslip via capillary action, eliminating air bubbles.

Gently heat the slide, preferably with an alcohol lamp or by other means, which does not leave too much soot under the glass slide (be sure to avoid boiling the content). Allow the specimen to stand for 15 to 30 minutes before examining it under a microscope. Examine for hyphae, spores, and budding cells.

Nail: Place several thin slices of nail shavings on a glass slide and cover with a coverslip. Since the most common type of onychomycosis involves subungual hyperkeratosis, a specimen from the subungual debris is preferred. Add several drops of KOH 10% to 30% solution at the edge of the coverslip, and the solution will be drawn under the coverslip via capillary action, eliminating air bubbles. Gently heat the slide, preferably with an alcohol lamp or by other means, which does not leave too much soot under the glass slide (be sure to avoid boiling the content). Allow the specimen to stand for 30 minutes before examining it under a microscope. The specimen should be examined for hyphae and budding cells.

Tzanck Smear

Although the viral culture remains the definitive test of herpes simplex infection, the Tzanck smear is a quick test that can be done in the office to help the physician make management decisions while the culture is pending. The Tzanck smear detects herpes simplex, herpes zoster, and varicella infections.

Vesicles are unroofed with a scalpel, and the vesicular fluid is collected and smeared onto a glass slide. Allow the content to air dry on the slide and then stain it with Wright's or Giemsa stain. Multinucleated giant cells seen under the microscope are pathognomonic for viral infections.

Dermatologic Therapy

Topical corticosteroids are the most frequently pre-scribed topical medications in dermatology. They are used for their antipruritic and anti-inflammatory effects. The mechanism of action of topical corticosteroids is complex and not thoroughly understood.

Topical corticosteroids are available in a range of different strengths ranked from group I through VII (see Appendix). Group I is the highest potency, and group VII is the lowest. Group VII topical corticosteroids are composed of drugs such as over-the-counter hydrocortisone 0.5% and 1%. The same preparation tends to be more potent in an ointment base than in a cream base because of the mild occlusive effect of the ointment, which enhances percutaneous penetration. For example, betamethasone dipropionate is available in a cream base as a group III topical corticosteroid (cream 0.05%) and in an ointment base as a group II topical corticosteroid (ointment 0.05%). Additionally, there are special formulations that enhance the percutaneous absorption and the potency of the topical corticosteroid. For example, the same betamethasone dipropionate is available as a group I topical corticosteroid (Diprolene®, ointment 0.05%). The exact concentration of topical corticosteroid is relevant only when comparing the same compound. For example, triamcinolone acetonide 0.1% ointment (Kenalog®) is stronger than its 0.025% cream formulation, but hydrocortisone 1% cream is much weaker than triamcinolone acetonide 0.025% cream.

Guidelines for Topical Corticosteroid Use

In prescribing a topical corticosteroid, several factors should be considered before making the selection—the potency, the agent, and the amount to be dispensed. Low-potency topical corticosteroids are recommended for dermatoses that are mild and chronic. Medium- and high-potency topical corticosteroids are used for dermatoses that are more severe or recalcitrant to treatment with weaker topical corticosteroids. Additionally, try to restrict topical corticosteroid use on the face and the intertriginous areas (ie, axilla, submammary, groin) to low-potency group VI or VII topical corticosteroids because they are less likely to cause local adverse effects. The face and the intertriginous areas are particularly prone to skin atrophy, which includes the formation of permanent stretch marks.

After the appropriate potency has been selected, the agent should be chosen. The vehicle is nearly as important as the active agent in the formulation of topical medications because the release of drugs varies greatly with different agents. The frequently used agents are creams, ointments, lotions, solutions, and gels. Creams (water-based) are white, nongreasy, and vanish when rubbed into the skin. Ointments (oil-based) are clear, greasy, and do not rub in when applied to the skin. Lotions are suspensions of powder in water, which evaporates to leave the active agent on the skin. Solutions are clear counterparts to lotions. Gels are transparent and colorless semisolid emulsions that liquefy when applied to the skin.

'Wet' cutaneous inflammations characterized by vesiculation, weeping, and crusting are best treated with nonocclusive agents such as cream, gel, or lotion. Ointment medications are best used on dry skin rashes. The greasy ointment film is lubricating and enhances penetration of the active ingredient through a mild occlusive effect. They are less acceptable aesthetically, however, because of their greasy nature. This is important because the patients' compliance is often directly related to their preference of agent; greasy ointments on the face and hands may be unacceptable to patients and may soak through clothing. We often recommend that patients use cream in the morning for elegance and ointment at bedtime for better efficacy and lubrication. For hairy areas, such as the scalp, lotions, solutions, or gels are best because they do not make these areas appear greasy.

Probably the most frequent error in prescribing a topical medication is the volume of medication dispensed. One gram of cream or ointment will cover an area approximately 10 cm x 10 cm. A single application of a cream or ointment to the face or hands requires 2 g; for 1 arm or the anterior

Table 1-7: Topical Corticosteroid Dose Needed for Single Application

Area	Dose
Face	2 g
Hands	2 g
One arm	3 g
One side of trunk	3 g
One leg	4 g
Whole body	30 g

or posterior trunk, 3 g; for 1 leg, 4 g; and for the entire body, 30 g (Table 1-7).

Clinicians have observed that chronic dermatoses, especially psoriasis, become less responsive after prolonged use of topical corticosteroids. This phenomenon is called tachyphylaxis.

Side Effects

Many side effects are associated with the use of topical corticosteroids (Table 1-8). Generally, the more potent the corticosteroid, the greater the likelihood of an adverse reaction. The most common side effect of topical corticosteroids is skin atrophy, manifested by thin, shiny, 'cigarette paper'-like skin; telangiectasia; and striae formation (stretch marks) (Figure 1-1; see color plate insert). Striae formation is permanent. Severe skin atrophy can lead to skin erosions. The face and intertriginous areas (ie, axilla, submammary, groin) are particularly prone to skin atrophy. The use of fluorinated corticosteroids (most topical corticosteroids other than hydrocortisone are fluorinated) can also cause corticosteroid acne in addition to skin atrophy.

Table 1-8: Side Effects of Topical Corticosteroids

Local
- Skin atrophy
- Acne
- Enhanced fungal skin infection
- Retarded wound and ulcer healing
- Contact dermatitis
- Glaucoma, cataracts (if used extensively around the eyes)

Systemic
- Adrenal suppression
- Cushing's syndrome
- Growth retardation in children

Additionally, topical corticosteroids may promote dermatophyte infections. They may also retard wound and ulcer healing and should not be used on these lesions. Allergic contact dermatitis sometimes occurs as a reaction to the agent or, even less often, to the topical corticosteroid itself. Allergic contact dermatitis should be suspected when the patient's skin condition is made worse by a topical corticosteroid. Cataracts and glaucoma have rarely been reported in association with extensive application of topical corticosteroids to the periorbital areas.

Systemic side effects (ie, adrenal suppression, Cushing's syndrome, growth retardation in children) from the use of topical corticosteroids are rare. These complications have been reported with extensive chronic use of potent topical corticosteroids, particularly when used under occlusion. The introduction of superpotent group I topical corticosteroids has increased the possibility of hypothalamic/ pituitary (HP) axis suppression. These superpotent group I topical corticosteroids generally should not be used for longer than 2 consecutive weeks, and the total dosage should not exceed 50 g/wk.

Cryosurgery

Keratoses and warts are frequently treated with liquid nitrogen cryosurgery. Liquid nitrogen is applied to the lesion with a cotton-tipped stick or directly with a spray and usually requires <30 seconds. A repeat freeze/thaw cycle results in more cellular damage than a single cycle.

During the procedure, the patient may feel a stinging or burning sensation. Subsequently, tissue swelling occurs. Usually, within 24 hours, a blister forms in the treated area and is allowed to crust spontaneously. If the blister is excessively large or painful, the fluid should be removed in a sterile manner.

Chapter 2

Papulosquamous Disorders

Psoriasis

Psoriasis is a set of heterogeneous genetic disorders that lead to a shortening of the keratinocyte cell cycle from 311 to 36 hours. As a result, keratinocytes proliferate at 28 times the normal rate, leading to pathognomonic plaque lesions that characterize the disease. Psoriasis affects 1% to 3% of the general population with equal incidence between genders. Psoriasis is an immune-mediated disorder; 5% to 8% of patients also experience psoriatic arthritis, a seronegative spondyloarthropathy. Heredity is a predictor in developing the disorder, with an 8% incidence when

---

Table 2-1: Trigger Factors for Psoriatic Flares

- Koebner's phenomenon: physical trauma, scarring, chronic rubbing, and scratching

- Drugs: systemic corticosteroid withdrawals, lithium, β-blockers, antimalarials, or interferon

- Infection: acute group A β-hemolytic streptococcal infection induces guttate psoriasis

- Stress

- Winter weather

Table 2-2: Treatment Options for Psoriasis

- Topical agents
  -corticosteroids
  -tar
  -anthralin (Psoriatec™)
   calcipotriene (Dovonex®)
  -tazarotene (Tazorac®)
  -betamethasone dipropionate/calcipotriene combination ointment (Taclonex®)

- Light therapy
  -broadband ultraviolet light B
  -narrowband UVB
  -psoralen/ultraviolet light A (PUVA)

- Oral agents
  -acitretin (Soriatane®)
  -cyclosporine
  -methotrexate

- Biologics
  -alefacept (Amevive®)
  -efalizumab (Raptiva®)
  -etanercept (Enbrel®)
  -adalimumab (Humira®)
  -infliximab (Remicade®)

one parent is affected and a 41% incidence when both parents are affected. Physiologic and environmental changes can trigger psoriasis. Trigger factors for psoriatic flares are listed in Table 2-1, and stress and winter weather are the most commonly reported trigger factors. Table 2-2 summarizes the treatment options for psoriasis.

Localized Plaque Psoriasis

Clinical diagnosis: Localized plaque psoriasis presents as well-demarcated erythematous plaques with characteristic silvery micaceous scale build-up (Figures 2-1 and 2-2; see color plate insert). Plaques are generally localized to extensor surfaces (ie, elbows, knees), although they can affect all areas of the body. Removal of the scales may lead to superficial bleeding in the area (Auspitz sign).

Treatment: Strong topical corticosteroids are the best choice for short-term use because they induce a fast response with minimal risk of irritation. Corticosteroids have serious shortcomings and liabilities over the long term, however, including the risk of skin atrophy with irreversible stretch mark formation, tachyphylaxis, and possible rebound phenomenon, in which the condition becomes worse than pretreatment after the medication is discontinued. Therefore, for long-term control of localized psoriasis, the use of noncorticosteroidal alternatives is preferred. Dermatologists often treat psoriasis in a sequential therapy mode (Table 2-3), which maximizes the initial speed of improvement using topical corticosteroids and provides a smooth transition to noncorticosteroid maintenance.

Class I corticosteroids are used to treat an acute flare. They should be applied twice daily to affected areas, and the patient must be followed closely (every 2 weeks) to monitor for signs of skin atrophy. Corticosteroids are contraindicated on the face, axillae, and groin because of the risk of skin atrophy. Continuous use of many superpotent topical corticosteroids is limited to 2 weeks at a time, according to the US Food and Drug Administration (FDA) guidelines.

Less-potent corticosteroids can be used for maintenance, including triamcinolone acetonide (Kenalog®) ointment used b.i.d. for the body; and desonide (DesOwen®) or alclometasone dipropionate (Aclovate®) used b.i.d. on the

Table 2-3: Topical Sequential Therapy of Psoriasis

Step I – Clearing phase (2-4 weeks)

q.a.m.	halobetasol (Ultravate®) cream*
q.h.s.	calcipotriene ointment

Step II – Transitional phase (4 weeks or longer)

weekdays b.i.d.	calcipotriene ointment
weekends b.i.d.	halobetasol cream*

Step III – Maintenance phase (up to 1 year)

b.i.d.	calcipotriene

* Generic clobetasol cream can be substituted if necessary.

face, axillae, and groin. The patient must be monitored closely for signs of skin atrophy.

A modified vitamin D topical agent, known as calcipotriene (Dovonex®), is the most widely used alternative to topical corticosteroids. It is more effective and less irritating than the vitamin A derivative, tazarotene (Tazorac®), and does not stain like tar or anthralin.

Calcipotriene is applied twice daily to affected areas. This regimen proved to be more effective than the steroid medication fluocinonide 0.05% (Lidex®) in a randomized, double-blind, controlled study.[1] Calcipotriene can be applied to all areas of the body without risk of skin atrophy. Its use should be limited to 100 g/wk to avoid the risk of hypercalcinosis. It has proven to be chemically compatible with the topical corticosteroid halobetasol propionate (Ultravate®) for a few days when freshly mixed and applied together.

Tazarotene 0.1% or 0.05% is a category X medication, which is contraindicated during pregancy; therefore, pregnancy prevention is required during its use by females of reproductive age. Tazarotene is applied nightly to affected areas. It offers a somewhat higher duration of remission than other topical agents, but tends to be significantly more irritating. Tazarotene should be applied sparingly only to psoriatic plaques and be discontinued at once if irritation occurs. Concurrent use of a topical corticosteroid every morning for at least 2 to 4 weeks is recommended for synergistic effectiveness and reduction of irritation. Mometasone furoate (Elocon®) cream has demonstrated a synergistic effect when used with tazarotene.[2]

Anthralin is applied q.d. to affected areas for 30 minutes to 1 hour and then washed off. Anthralin has been used to treat psoriasis for more than 100 years, but its tendency to stain clothing and linens is a drawback.

Coal tar is applied q.d. to affected areas. It is safe for long-term use.

Corticosteroid intralesional injections, such as triamcinolone acetonide aqueous suspension (Kenalog-10®, Kenalog-40®) 10 mg/mL and 40 mg/mL, respectively, are useful for treating small plaques (<4 cm). They are injected superficially and intradermally, requiring some pressure to push the medicine into the psoriatic plaques. Injections without resistance indicate an incorrect injection into subcutaneous space.

Generalized Plaque Psoriasis

Clinical diagnosis: Generalized plaque psoriasis appears the same as localized plaque psoriasis, except for the appearance of confluent plaques throughout the body (Figure 2-3; see color plate insert).

Treatment: Topical treatment alone is usually inadequate because of the large areas of involvement. Systemic therapy and phototherapy are the primary treatment modalities, and treatment should be: (1) managed by an experienced dermatologist who has access to phototherapy units, or (2) provided in a specialized psoriasis day-care treatment center. Systemic agents include oral retinoids such as acitretin (Soriatane®), methotrexate (Rheumatrex®, Trexall™), and cyclosporine (Neoral®). Phototherapy options include psoralen/ultraviolet light A (PUVA) (oral 8-methoxypsoralen [8-MOP®, Oxsoralen-Ultra®] followed by ultraviolet light A and ultraviolet light B). Specialized centers can also provide Goeckerman therapy (tar and UVB combination therapy).

The following list of oral agents is provided to familiarize clinicians with commonly used and FDA-approved oral agents for psoriasis and is not meant to be a comprehensive guideline for their use.

Oral retinoids (acitretin): Dosage is usually 25 mg to 50 mg q.d., with food. Treatment should be started on the second or third day of the menstrual period in women of reproductive age.

Monitoring:
- Baseline: pregnancy test; complete blood count (CBC), aspartate aminotransferase (AST), and fasting lipid panel (total cholesterol, triglycerides, low-density lipoprotein [LDL], high-density lipoprotein [HDL]).
- Biweekly, until stabilized: CBC, AST, and fasting lipid panel (total cholesterol, triglycerides, LDL, HDL).
- Monthly: pregnancy test, CBC, AST, and fasting lipid panel (total cholesterol, triglycerides, LDL, HDL).
- Posttreatment: monthly pregnancy test until 1 year posttreatment.

Precautions: Oral retinoids are category X medications. For menstruating women, two forms of birth control should be started 1 month before treatment and continued until 3 years posttreatment. Pregnancy must be avoided until 3 years posttreatment. Acitretin interferes with the oral progestin 'minipill.' Drinking milk increases absorption, and vitamin A may increase its toxicity. Ethanol increases the drug's half-life and must be avoided by women until 2 months posttreatment. Taking tetracycline can increase the incidence of pseudotumor cerebri. Patients should not make blood donations for 3 years posttreatment.

Methotrexate: The usual effective dose is 15 mg/wk, to a maximum of 30 mg/wk. One test dose of 5 mg is given to check for sensitivity. Divided dosing (2.5 mg q12h x 3 doses) is recommended to reduce gastrointestinal (GI) upset.

Monitoring:
- Baseline: liver function tests (LFT), blood urea nitrogen (BUN), creatinine, CBC with differential.
- One week after test dose: LFT, CBC with differential.
- Monthly: LFT, BUN, creatinine, CBC with differential.
- Liver biopsy after the first 1.5 g of methotrexate, then at a cumulative dose of 3 g, and then every 1 g thereafter.

Precautions: Methotrexate is a category X medication. Contraception for men and women is required during treatment and for 3 months posttreatment. Its use is contraindicated in the presence of liver disease or alcohol use. It has 10 black box warnings, including possible increased risk of lymphoma, pneumonitis, and GI ulcerations.

Cyclosporine: Dosage is 2.5 mg/kg/d to 4 mg/kg/d divided b.i.d. dosing. Start at 2.5 mg/kg/d for 4 weeks; increase by 0.5 mg/kg/d every 2 weeks until clinical response is achieved. Discontinue use if it is not effective at 4 mg/kg/d after 6 weeks. Continuous use is recommended for 1 year. The patient must be off the medication for several months before restarting cyclosporine.

Monitoring:
- Baseline: fasting cholesterol panel (triglycerides, LDL, HDL), CBC, BUN, creatinine, LFT, magnesium, potassium, and two normal blood pressure readings.
- Biweekly for 3 months: fasting cholesterol panel (triglycerides, LDL, HDL), CBC, BUN, creatinine, LFT, and magnesium.
- Monthly: fasting cholesterol panel (triglycerides, LDL, HDL), CBC, BUN, creatinine, LFT, and magnesium.
- A 30% increase in creatinine must be followed by a 25% decrease in dose.

Precautions: Cyclosporine is contraindicated in patients with hypertension, malignancy, and abnormal renal function.

Biologic Agents for Treating Psoriasis

The following list of biologic agents is provided to familiarize clinicians with FDA-approved treatments for psoriasis and is not meant to be a comprehensive guideline for their use.

Alefacept: Alefacept (Amevive®) is a fusion protein combining a portion of human immunoglobulin G (IgG) and the binding site of lymphocyte function-associated antigen-3 (LFA-3). It binds to CD2, the partner molecule of LFA-3 located on the surface of T cells. This drug also binds to the surface proteins of accessory cells, including natural killer cells and macrophages. Alefacept inhibits T-cell activation and proliferation and also induces T-cell apoptosis. Because it depletes a subset of CD4 T cells, the absolute CD4 count may decline and must be monitored during treatment.

Alefacept is administered via intramuscular (IM) injection. A dosing course consists of 12 weekly administrations of 15 mg IM. Absolute CD4 counts must be performed every other week during treatment, and the dose must be held if the CD4 count drops below 250 cells/mm³. Onset of action is slow, and patients typically continue to exhibit improvement even after the last dose of a course. Patients can repeat courses of alefacept, as long as their CD4 counts are within normal range and at least 12 weeks have elapsed between courses.

Efalizumab: Efalizumab (Raptiva®) is a humanized monoclonal antibody directed against the T-cell surface molecule CD11a. CD11a and CD18 proteins form lymphocyte function-associated antigen-1 (LFA-1), which plays a critical role in allowing lymphocytes to adhere to other cell types. Binding of efalizumab to CD11a blocks the interaction between LFA-1 and intracellular adhesion molecule-1 (ICAM-1), its partner molecule on the surface of antigen-presenting cells (APCs), vascular endothelial cells, and keratinocytes. Psoriasis-inducing T cells are thereby prevented from being activated in the lymph nodes or reactivated in the dermis and epidermis. ICAM-1's presence on endothelial cells also prevents T cells blocked by efalizumab from binding to the blood vessel wall and migrating into the skin.

Efalizumab is available as a subcutaneous (SC) preparation that patients can self-inject once weekly. The recommended dose is a single 0.7 mg/kg SC conditioning dose followed by weekly SC doses of 1 mg/kg, maximum dose not to exceed 200 mg. Dosing can be continuous with a good durability of response.

Etanercept: Tumor necrosis factor-α (TNF-α) is a pro-inflammatory cytokine found in increased concentrations in the joints and skin in psoriatic arthritis and psoriasis, respectively. Endogenous skin cells and activated leukocytes secrete TNF-α, which binds to target receptors that are found on almost every cell in the body. Tumor necrosis factor plays an active role in leukocyte recruitment, migration, and activation. Leukocytes activated by TNF secrete more cytokines, creating an inflammatory cascade.

Etanercept (Enbrel®) is a fusion protein consisting of two TNF receptors fused to the Fc portion of human IgG antibody. This construct creates an exogenous TNF receptor and prevents excess TNF from binding to cell-bound receptors. The end result is a reduction of active TNF and mitigation of diseases, such as rheumatoid arthritis and psoriasis, that are mediated by the effects of TNF.

Enbrel® is available as a SC preparation that patients can self-inject, 50 mg once or twice weekly. Dosing can be continuous with good durability of response.

Infliximab: Similar to efalizumab, infliximab (Remicade®) is a monoclonal antibody, but this drug targets TNF and is administered intravenously. An initial infusion of 5 mg/kg is given, followed by repeat administrations 2 and 6 weeks later. Patients can then be maintained with an infusion every 2 months.

Screening for tuberculosis (TB) before starting therapy is particularly important because infliximab has been associated with rare incidents of reactivation of TB in patients with latent infection.

Guttate Psoriasis

Clinical diagnosis: This distinctive form of psoriasis often follows acute group A β-hemolytic streptococcal pharyngitis. Guttate psoriasis usually occurs in patients <30 years of age. Lesions are numerous, generalized erythematous papules 2 to 5 mm in diameter distributed throughout the body. Later, they can become confluent plaques with relative sparing of the palms and soles. A throat culture should be taken to rule out group A β-hemolytic streptococcal infection. Serum antistreptolysin (ASO) titers may be elevated.

Antistreptococcal oral antibiotics (eg, penicillin) may be indicated. Guttate psoriasis is also usually rapidly responsive to topical steroids or ultraviolet light B phototherapy.

Treatment: Guttate psoriasis may resolve spontaneously after a treatment course of several weeks. Persistent cases are treated as in generalized plaque psoriasis.

Scalp Psoriasis

Clinical diagnosis: Psoriatic plaques on the scalp sometimes resemble seborrheic dermatitis. Generally, scalp psoriasis appears as well-demarcated silvery plaques with mild induration and erythema; seborrheic dermatitis is usually poorly demarcated and diffuse. Although usually asymptomatic, scalp psoriasis may be extremely pruritic, but lesions usually do not scar or cause alopecia.

Treatment: If the patient has thick scales, they can be removed with fluocinolone acetonide 0.01% oil (Derma-Smoothe/FS®). This step is optional. Once scales are removed, topical corticosteroid lotions, gels, or solutions are used for thick plaques. Topical corticosteroid in foam formulation, such as betamethasone valerate (Luxiq®) or clobetasol propionate (Olux®), provide a cosmetically elegant treatment for the scalp. Although skin atrophy of the scalp is unlikely, patients should nevertheless be warned not to use Class I corticosteroids for >2 weeks continuously as a general rule of thumb. Calcipotriene solution may be used as combination therapy in addition to topical corticosteroid and as maintenance treatment.

Nail Psoriasis

Clinical diagnosis: Characteristic changes in fingernails and toenails include pitting, subungual hyperkeratosis, onycholysis, and pathognomonic 'oil spots' (yellowish-brown spots underneath the nail plate).

Treatment: Because of the poor absorption of medications into the nail beds, topical treatment of nails is usually unsatisfactory. Intralesional corticosteroid injections of triamcinolone acetonide (Kenalog-10®, Kenalog-40®) at approximately 3 mg/mL may be helpful, but they are painful and can cause hemorrhaging under the nail plate.

Localized and Generalized Acute Pustular Psoriasis

Generalized pustular psoriasis is one of the rare, life-threatening dermatologic emergencies where a patient needs to be promptly hospitalized for intensive monitoring. Localized pustular psoriasis is often debilitating but is not usually life-threatening (Figure 2-4; see color plate insert). There may or may not be a history of plaque psoriasis. In the United States, one of the more common precipitating factors for acute generalized pustular psoriasis is a withdrawal reaction from systemic corticosteroids used to treat psoriasis. Because of this risk of pustular conversion where plaque-type psoriasis becomes pustular, the use of systemic corticosteroids to treat psoriasis is generally discouraged except when there is no other alternative.

Clinical diagnosis: The patient starts out with generalized erythroderma of acute onset. Characteristic nonfol-

Table 2-4: Treatment for Generalized Acute Pustular Psoriasis

- Acute hospitalization is necessary, and patient is managed as extensive-burn patient.
- Blood cultures should be taken if bacterial sepsis and/or superinfection are suspected.
- Intravenous fluids are necessary to avoid dehydration.
- Administering antibiotics is prudent until bacterial infections are ruled out.
- In-patient dermatologic care supervised by a dermatologist is critical.
- Patient must be closely monitored for any sign of infection.
- Oral retinoid, cyclosporine, and/or methotrexate may be required.

licular pinpoint pustules then appear in clusters and may coalesce into small pools filled with purulent fluid. The evolution of this clinical picture is so rapid that it may appear within a single day. Patients generally present with tachycardia, tachypnea, and fever, resembling a septic picture, which may evolve to a life-threatening septic state.

Treatment: Acute hospitalization is necessary, and the patient is managed as an extensive-burn patient. Blood cultures should be taken if bacterial sepsis and/or superinfection are suspected. Intravenous fluids are important to avoid dehydration, and administering antibiotics is prudent until bacterial infections are ruled out. In-patient dermatologic care supervised by a dermatologist is critical. The patient must be closely monitored for any sign of infection. Oral retinoid, cyclosporine, or methotrexate may be required (Table 2-4).

Seborrheic Dermatitis

Seborrheic dermatitis (SD)—including seborrhea, cradle cap (in infants), pityriasis sicca (dandruff), and eczematoid seborrhea—is a common chronic inflammatory scaling condition associated with increased rates of maturation and proliferation of epidermal cells with variable retention of sebum. *Pityrosporum ovale*, a fungus, is thought to play a role. The condition affects all age groups (with the exception of cradle cap, which occurs in infants) and is more prevalent in males and older populations. Patients with HIV have a higher prevalence of SD.

Clinical diagnosis: Seborrheic dermatitis presents as poorly demarcated areas of mild erythema and greasy white to yellow scales and variable pruritus. The distribution of scales often follows areas of sebaceous glands, such as the scalp, eyebrows, eyelashes, beard, forehead, nasolabial folds, glabella, upper midback, sternum, axillae, groin, and anogenital areas. Common differential diagnosis includes psoriasis vulgaris, impetigo, fungal infections, and tinea versicolor.

Treatment: Seborrheic dermatitis is a chronic disease that requires initial therapy followed by maintenance therapy. A variety of over-the-counter shampoos are effective for treating SD. The shampoos can be used on the scalp and any other areas of the body that are affected; they are used daily until the condition is brought under control, after which they should be used only once to twice weekly for maintenance. Mild SD can be treated with shampoos containing tar, selenium sulfide (Selsun®), or zinc pyrithione (Head & Shoulders®). Moderate-to-severe SD often responds to shampoos or creams containing 2% ketoconazole (Nizoral®), used daily until it is under control, then once to twice weekly for maintenance. Low-potency topical corticosteroids (1% to 2.5% hydro-

Table 2-5: Treatment for Seborrheic Dermatitis

Mild

- Shampoos containing tar, selenium sulfide, or zinc pyrithione daily until under control, then once to twice weekly for maintenance.

Moderate to Severe

- Shampoos/creams containing 2% ketoconazole (Nizoral®) daily until under control, then once to twice weekly for maintenance.

- Low-potency corticosteroids (1% to 2.5% hydrocortisone) or stronger corticosteroids, such as desonide (DesOwen®) or alclometasone dipropionate (Aclovate®), may be used initially but not as maintenance therapy.

---

cortisone) or stronger corticosteroids, such as desonide or alclometasone dipropionate, may be used initially but not as maintenance therapy (Table 2-5).

Patients with seborrheic blepharitis are more difficult to treat and may need a referral to an ophthalmologist.

Pityriasis Rosea

Pityriasis rosea is an acute, self-limiting, inflammatory dermatosis that primarily affects older children and young adults. It is clinically characterized by oval, fawn-colored (pink-tan), minimally elevated, scaling patches, papules, and plaques that are primarily located on the trunk. The exact cause is unknown, but a viral etiology has been suspected.

Clinical diagnosis: Characteristically, most patients develop one large (1 to 10 cm) patch, which is called the 'herald patch,' before the others. After several days, numerous smaller patches appear, mainly on the trunk and proximal parts of the extremities. They are typically oval, faint pink, with a collarette of delicate scales well inside the border of the lesion. On the back, longitudinal axes of the lesions run down and out relative to the spine in a pattern that, with imagination, has been likened to a Christmas tree. The patient usually feels well, but itching often occurs and ranges in severity from mild to moderate.

Because secondary syphilis can mimic pityriasis rosea closely, a serologic test for syphilis should be ordered in all cases of 'atypical' pityriasis rosea, eg, if there is no herald patch, if the distal extremities (especially the palms and soles) are involved, or if the patient is systemically ill.

Treatment: Offering the patient reassurance is usually all that is necessary for this self-limited disease. Anti-itch medications, ie, calamine lotion or oral antihistamines, may be prescribed if necessary. The eruption usually lasts between 2 and 10 weeks and then resolves spontaneously. The condition rarely recurs. There are usually no complications, except for occasional postinflammatory hypopigmentation or hyperpigmentation, which resolves slowly over time, often months.

References

1.   Bruce S, Epinette WW, Funicella T, et al: Comparative study of calcipotriene (MC 903) ointment and fluocinonide ointment in the treatment of psoriasis. *J Am Acad Dermatol* 1994;31(5 pt 1):755-759.

2.   Lebwohl MG, Breneman DL, Goffe BS, et al: Tazarotene 0.1% gel plus corticosteroid cream in the treatment of plaque psoriasis. *J Am Acad Dermatol* 1998;39(4 pt 1):590-596.

Chapter 3

Eczematous Dermatitis

Atopic Dermatitis

Atopic dermatitis is a chronic, pruritic rash that is caused by an overactive or misguided immune system (Figure 3-1; see color plate insert). It is often associated with a personal or family history of atopic disease (eg, asthma, allergic rhinitis). The skin of patients with atopic dermatitis is in a state of hyperirritability, and itching is the primary symptom. Because of the itching, patients scratch and the skin becomes excoriated. Excoriation exacerbates the itching and, therefore, perpetuates the itch/scratch cycle, maintaining the state of inflammation. There appears to be a genetic predisposition for atopic dermatitis that can be affected by numerous factors, including food allergies, skin infections, irritating clothes (ie, wool), chemicals, and emotional stress. Many doctors refer to this condition as eczema or 'the itch that rashes.'

Atopic dermatitis is predominantly a disease of child-hood and young adulthood, with 5% of children affected. It usually starts after 2 months of age, and by 5 years of age, 90% of the patients who will develop atopic dermatitis have manifested the disease. Most children (90%) outgrow it by adolescence, although as adults, some will continue to have localized forms of eczema (Figure 3-2; see color plate insert), such as chronic hand or foot dermatitis, patches of lichen simplex chronicus, or eyelid dermatitis. It is uncommon for adults to develop atopic dermatitis without a history of childhood eczema.

Clinical diagnosis: The clinical findings of atopic dermatitis are often divided into acute and chronic categories. The acute stage starts out with itching and flat erythematous patches on the skin. Because of the skin's inflammatory reaction, infiltration and papulation may occur. In severe acute cases, vesiculation of the skin and leaking of fluid or exudative-type lesions on excoriation may occur. As the lesions become more chronic and are continually scratched by the patient, the eczema becomes leathery and dry. The skin becomes thickened with accentuated skin lines (lichenification). Certain patients with prolonged scratching in specific areas develop prurigo lesions, which are nodules that appear on the skin as the result of chronic scratching.

The distribution of atopic dermatitis changes depending on the patient's age. In infancy and early childhood, the face is the most common site of involvement. In later childhood, adolescence, and adulthood, a shift occurs from the face to the flexural surfaces, usually affecting the antecubital and popliteal fossae, wrists, and ankles, but not the face.

Patients with atopic dermatitis exhibit a number of immunologic abnormalities. They tend to have an overactivity of T cells, specifically T-helper type 2 (Th_2) cells vs T-helper type 1 (Th_1) cells. T-helper type 2 cells are often associated with increasing or encouraging the humoral immune system to elaborate immunoglobulin E (IgE), so elevated IgE levels are common in these patients.

Treatment: The treatment goal in acute atopic dermatitis is to decrease the itching and/or scratching so that the skin can gradually heal. Management of mild atopic dermatitis may simply consist of good skin care: good skin hydration and liberal use of emollients after showering or bathing to help maintain the hydrated state of the skin. Even humidifiers in the home will help some patients. The key is that these patients have irritable skin that reacts to often nonspecific stimuli, which include chronic xerosis (dryness or dehydration). Moisturizers reduce dry skin and itching.

Table 3-1: Exacerbating Factors for Eczema

- Anxiety or stress
- Climatic factors
  - temperature
  - humidity
- Irritants
  - detergents, solvents
  - wool or other rough material
- Food, contact, or inhaled antigens

If patients can identify factors that cause their eczema to worsen, they can avoid exposure to these factors (Table 3-1). Patients often notice their disease gets worse during periods of anxiety and stress. Climatic factors, such as extremes of temperature, low humidity (which decreases skin hydration), and, in some patients, high humidity (which causes sweating), can make the disease worse. Patients should use mild soaps or soap substitutes because detergents, soaps, and solvents may be irritating and excessively drying. Wool clothing is often irritating to these patients. Some atopic patients may experience worsening symptoms from food or aeroallergens that they inhale or that come into contact with their skin. Commonly implicated foods are eggs, milk, shellfish, strawberries, citrus fruit, peanuts, other nuts, wheat, and fish.

Immunomodulatory therapy is the mainstay of treatment for atopic dermatitis (Table 3-2). Corticosteroids are the most widely prescribed medications to control atopic dermatitis. Corticosteroids can be used topically or systemically, but ointments are usually preferable since they are significant emollients that deliver the corticosteroid in

Table 3-2: Atopic Dermatitis Management

- Skin hydration
  - emollients
- Immunomodulatory therapy
  - pimecrolimus (Elidel®)
  - tacrolimus (Protopic®)
  - corticosteroids
  - ultraviolet light B or psoralen/ultraviolet light A (PUVA) phototherapy
  - cyclosporine (Neoral®)
- Antihistamines for pruritus
- Antistaphylococcal oral antibiotics (dicloxacillin, cephalexin [Keflex®])
- Avoidance of exacerbating factors

a more efficient manner. Further details on corticosteroids can be found in Chapter 1. Some patients with severe or recalcitrant disease may require systemic corticosteroid treatment. These patients may benefit from a referral to a dermatologist, who can confirm the diagnosis and evaluate whether other topical or systemic therapy for eczema would be more effective.

Tacrolimus (Protopic®) and pimecrolimus (Elidel®) are two nonsteroidal agents in a class of medications known as topical immunomodulators (TIMs). Topical immunomodulators are an effective and promising alternative to topical corticosteroids. Tacrolimus and pimecrolimus molecules are macrolides with a mechanism of action similar to the immunomodulator cyclosporine (Neoral®). They act as calcineurin inhibitors, inhibiting T-cell activation by blocking the transcription of early proinflammatory cytokines (ie, interleukin [IL]-2, interferon-γ, IL-4, and IL-10) as well as inhibiting mast cell degranulation.

Tacrolimus is available as Protopic® 0.1% and 0.03% ointment; both are indicated for b.i.d. treatment of moderate-to-severe atopic dermatitis. Protopic® 0.03% is approved for use in patients between 2 and 15 years of age, while Protopic® 0.1% is approved for use in patients older than 15 years. Pimecrolimus is available as Elidel® 1% cream, which is indicated for b.i.d. treatment of mild-to-moderate atopic dermatitis for patients 2 years or older. The foremost difference between these two agents is the vehicle of administration: pimecrolimus is a cream and tacrolimus is an ointment. The choice between the two is based, in part, on patient preference, which is an integral aspect of compliance. Generally, compliance is better with cream than with ointment, even though ointment may be more lubricating.

Primary care providers may be concerned about immunosuppression. However, manifestations of topical immunosuppression (ie, bacterial, viral, fungal, yeast superinfections) are not higher when these agents are compared with placebo. Furthermore, both agents, when applied topically, do not maintain blood levels that would cause systemic immunosuppression. The only documented cases of persistent systemic absorption occurred with the use of tacrolimus in Netherton's syndrome, which involves a congenital impairment of skin barrier function.

There is a black box warning on the package inserts for Elidel® and Protopic®. This decision by the US Food and Drug Administration (FDA) was based on the finding of a theoretic risk of lymphoma or nonmelanoma skin cancer from these medications based on animal models. The animal subjects were given large doses of the drugs orally or the drugs were applied topically in a vehicle that enhances penetration. Human studies have not substantiated an association between topical tacrolimus or pimecrolimus and cancers as of the publication of this handbook.

The American Academy of Dermatology (AAD) strongly maintains that these drugs are safe with proper use, and acknowledges that it is the physician's responsibility to inform and educate patients regarding the benefits and risks involved, and to monitor patients accordingly.

With the advent of nonsteroidal TIMs, the paradigm for treatment of atopic dermatitis should now focus on prevention and early treatment to minimize the use of topical corticosteroids. Patients with chronic atopic dermatitis can be treated with either pimecrolimus or tacrolimus as maintenance therapy, with topical corticosteroids added to the regimen during flare-up episodes when nonsteroidal TIM therapy proves inadequate. For patients with intermittent atopic dermatitis, pimecrolimus or tacrolimus can be used as a first-line 'controller' treatment, with topical corticosteroids reserved for short-term use during flare-up episodes inadequately controlled by nonsteroidal TIMs.

Ultraviolet light B or psoralen (8-MOP®, Oxsoralen-Ultra® [8-methoxypsoralen]) plus ultraviolet light A [PUVA]) may be considered if satisfactory control is not achieved with topical treatment. Cyclosporine is another alternative for patients with atopic dermatitis recalcitrant to topical treatments.

Skin infections by bacteria and viruses are more common in patients with atopic dermatitis. There is a higher rate of colonization with *Staphylococcus aureus* in involved and noninvolved skin in atopic dermatitis, and patients are more susceptible to staphylococcal infections or impetigo. Many patients benefit from antistaphylococcal antibiotics, even when clinical evidence of infection is lacking. Oral dicloxacillin at a dose of 125 mg to 500 mg 4 times daily or cephalexin (Keflex®) at a dose of 250 mg to 500 mg 4 times daily are common options. Eczema patients are also prone to cutaneous infections with viruses such as herpes and human papillomavirus; these patients are also more prone to warts and molluscum contagiosum. In addition, there is increased susceptibility to a generalized herpes simplex infection called eczema herpeticum, which presents as the sudden appearance of vesicular, pustular, crusted, or punched-out erosive lesions concentrated in the areas of dermatitis. In eczema herpeticum, secondary staphylococcal infection may occur. Systemic acyclovir (Zovirax®) and an antistaphylococcal antibiotic are recommended.

Atopic dermatitis is characterized by exacerbations and remissions. Patients will cycle from periods of flare-ups and extreme involvement to times when they essentially have a holiday from their disease. In most patients, the severity of disease decreases with age, even if it persists to some degree. Patients who have had the disease in childhood, although they may not have widespread atopic dermatitis as they grow older, are often more susceptible to conditions such as hand eczema, and allergic and irritant contact dermatitis from common irritants that might not bother a nonatopic patient.

Contact Dermatitis

Contact dermatitis is an inflammatory condition caused by exposure to allergens or irritant chemicals (Figures 3-3 and 3-4; see color plate insert). Contact dermatitis can be separated into two categories: 'true' allergic contact dermatitis and irritant dermatitis. Allergic contact dermatitis is a type IV hypersensitivity reaction, in which the clinical manifestations occur 24 to 72 hours after allergen exposure in previously sensitized persons. In contrast, irritant dermatitis requires no prior sensitization. When exposed to an adequate level of irritating chemicals, all people develop irritant toxic contact dermatitis after a few hours. The acute condition evolves into a chronic condition when exposure to the allergen or irritating chemical is repeated.

Clinical diagnosis: Acute contact dermatitis manifests first as erythema and scaling, which can progress to vesicles,

Table 3-3: Treatment for Contact Dermatitis

Localized/Mild

- Avoidance of allergen and irritant chemicals

- Group I topical corticosteroids such as augmented betamethasone (Diprolene®), clobetasol (Temovate®), diflorasone (Psorcon®), halobetasol (Ultravate®), and fluocinonide 0.1% (Vanos™)

Severe

- Intramuscular (IM) corticosteroids

- Oral prednisone, short course with a 2-week to 3-week taper

erosions, and finally to crusting. A rash caused by contact dermatitis as a result of irritant exposure tends to have a more clearly defined border. Contact dermatitis caused by allergen exposure initially has a clearly defined border that later may become obscured because of the cell-mediated immunologic nature of the reaction. Chronic contact dermatitis presents as crusty and scaly plaques with ill-defined borders.

Treatment: Localized contact dermatitis can be resolved through avoidance of allergen and irritant chemicals, and use of group I topical corticosteroids, (ie, augmented betamethasone [Diprolene®], clobetasol [Temovate®], diflorasone [Psorcon®], halobetasol [Ultravate®], fluocinonide 0.1% [Vanos™]). Severe cases may require IM corticosteroids, or a short course of oral prednisone with a 2-week to 3-week taper (Table 3-3). A course of oral prednisone with a 2-week to 3-week taper is particularly important in the treatment of allergic contact dermatitis, such as poison oak dermatitis, where effective control of the eruptions may be compromised with a too-short course of oral prednisone.

Table 3-4: Treatments for Lichen Simplex Chronicus

- Avoid scratching
- Intralesional corticosteroids
- High-potency topical corticosteroids

Lichen Simplex Chronicus

Clinical diagnosis: Lichen simplex chronicus (also called neurodermatitis) is a chronic pruritic eruption of the skin resulting from chronic scratching. It usually occurs as a single, fixed, lichenified (thickened skin with accentuated skin lines) plaque that is extremely pruritic. Itching typically precedes the scratching, although the rubbing and scratching is often unconscious, either as a habit or in response to emotional stress. The scratching then causes the lichenification, and the lichenified skin itself itches, resulting in an 'itch/scratch/itch' cycle that perpetuates the process.

Treatment: Patients should be reminded frequently to stop scratching and rubbing the skin. High-potency topical corticosteroids or intralesional corticosteroids are helpful to break the scratch/itch cycle (Table 3-4). Occlusion over topical corticosteroid greatly enhances the effectiveness of topical corticosteroids, as well as prevents scratching. For small lesions, flurandrenolide (Cordran®) tape, which incorporates corticosteroid into its adhesive, is beneficial because it protects the affected area from scratching as well as provides a superpotent topical corticosteroid.

Chapter 4

Pigmentary Disorders

Vitiligo

Vitiligo is an acquired condition in which melanocytes in affected skin are dysfunctional or have disappeared (Figure 4-1; see color plate insert). Lesions clinically appear as white, nonscaling, sharply demarcated macules or patches. Vitiligo is usually asymptomatic with most patients seeking medical help because of disfigurement. The disease begins at any age, but the peak incidence is in the 10- to 30-year-old age group. The exact cause is unknown, but an autoimmune mechanism has been suspected.

Vitiligo begins as one or more small white spots that gradually enlarge. Vitiligo can affect any area of the skin and mucous membranes, but the most common areas are the extensor bony surfaces (ie, knuckles, elbows, knees) and the periorificial areas (ie, around the mouth, eyes, rectum, genitalia). Involvement of hairy areas often results in depigmentation of the hair as well.

Clinical diagnosis: The lesions can be appreciated best by Wood's light examination, which accentuates the pigment contrast and makes evident previously undetected areas in patients with lightly pigmented skin. Thyroid function tests and a complete blood count (CBC) with differential may be ordered to screen for rarely associated thyroid disease and pernicious anemia, as well as Addison's disease.

Treatment: For limited disease, potent topical steroids may be effective in some patients when applied twice daily

Table 4-1: Treatments for Vitiligo

- Potent topical corticosteroids
- Skin dyes and cosmetics
- PUVA phototherapy
- Topical calcipotriene (Dovonex®)

for months (Table 4-1). Patients should be examined every 1 to 2 months for signs of skin atrophy from chronic topical steroid use. Recently, topical calcipotriene (Dovonex®) has been reported to be efficacious in some patients with vitiligo. Topical treatments for vitiligo are generally unreliable and have a low probability of success. If topical treatment fails, referral to a dermatologist is recommended. The only US Food and Drug Administration (FDA)-approved treatment for vitiligo is photochemotherapy with psoralen (8-methoxypsoralen [8-MOP®, Oxsoralen-Ultra®])/ultraviolet light A (PUVA). Narrowband ultraviolet light B phototherapy has been reported to be an effective and promising treatment for vitiligo and is more convenient compared with PUVA because patients do not have to take psoralen pills. Vitiligo burns easily in the sun; therefore, sun avoidance and the use of sunscreens are important to avoid sunburn of the affected areas.

Vitiligo is slow to respond to treatment, taking weeks to months before repigmentation occurs. It is important to encourage vitiligo sufferers to be patient. Complete repigmentation can be expected in 15% to 20% of cases, with 75% repigmentation in another 15%. There is no response in at least 20% of cases. Response is manifested by the development of enlarging pigmented spots in the center of the lesions or as irregular encroachments of pigment at the margins. Facial, neck, trunk, and genital lesions are the most

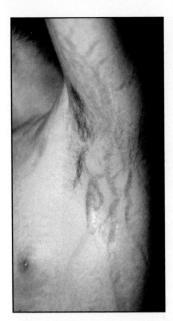

Figure 1-1: Skin atrophy caused by use of topical steroid.

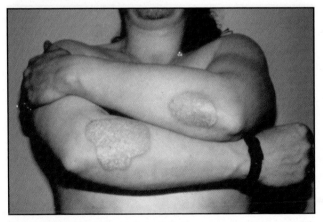

Figure 2-1: Psoriasis (localized).

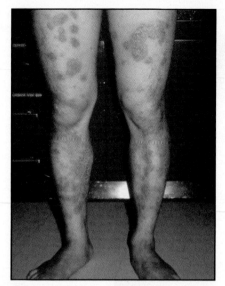

Figure 2-2: Psoriasis (moderate).

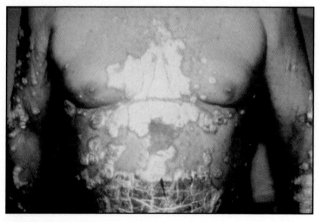

Figure 2-3: Psoriasis (severe).

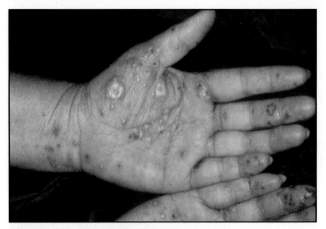

Figure 2-4: Pustular psoriasis.

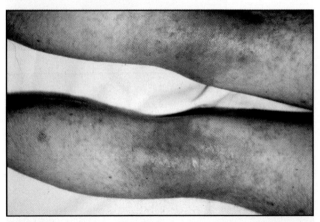

Figure 3-1: Atopic dermatitis.

Figure 3-2:
Eczema.

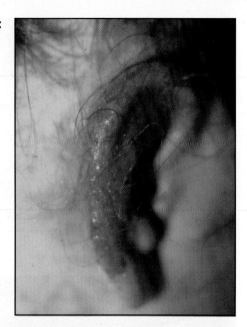

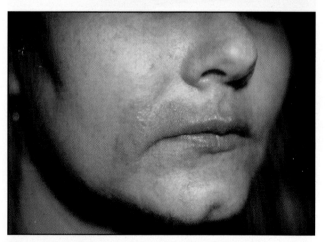

Figure 3-3: Contact dermatitis (food allergy).

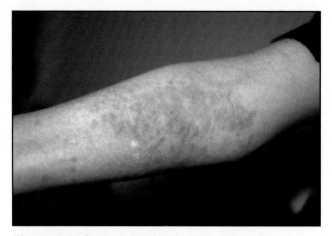

Figure 3-4: Contact dermatitis (drug allergy).

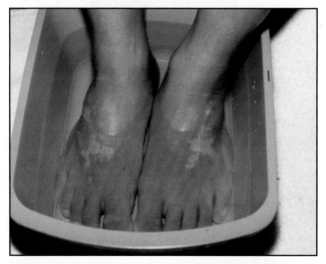

Figure 4-1: Vitiligo.

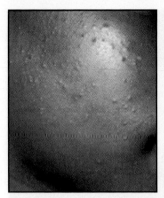

Figure 5-1: Mild acne.

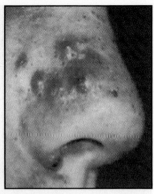

Figure 5-2: Moderate acne.

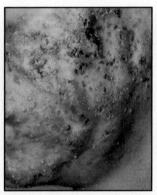

Figure 5-3: Severe acne.

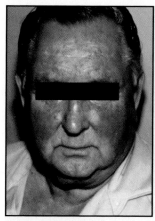

Figure 5-4: Rosacea.

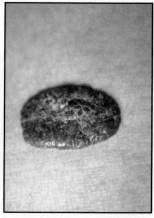

Figure 6-1: Seborrheic keratosis.

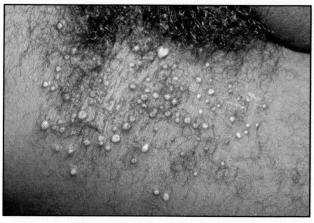

Figure 7-1: Folliculitis caused by *Staphylococcus aureus*.

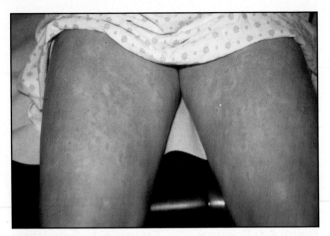

Figure 8-1: Urticaria.

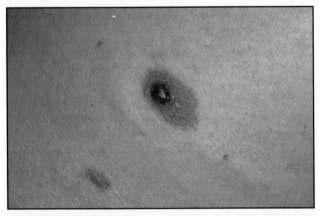

Figure 9-1: Nodular melanoma arising from a nevus.

responsive; lesions over joints and distal extremities are the least responsive to treatment. The most recent lesions tend to respond best. If there is no response after 3 months of treatment, then continuation of the same treatment is unlikely to work. Once repigmentation occurs, it usually persists. The patient may undergo as much as 2 years of treatment before the maximum benefit is reached.

An alternative to narrowband UVB or PUVA treatment is to cover the lesions with a cosmetic that is blended to match the color of the patient's normal skin. This approach is especially useful for small areas or on the eyelids, where potent topical steroids should not be used. Additionally, over-the-counter self-tanning cream may be applied on skin affected by vitiligo to soften the contrast between the depigmented and normal skin. Self-tanning creams tend to give more satisfactory response in lighter-complexioned persons than those with darker complexions.

The course of vitiligo is unpredictable. In most patients, it is chronic and often progresses slowly. Spontaneous repigmentation occurs in a minority of patients but usually is incomplete.

Melasma

Melasma is an acquired condition that causes patchy, irregular brown hyperpigmentation on the face. It occurs most frequently among pregnant women and those taking birth control pills. It is more common in patients with darker skin color.

Clinical diagnosis: Lesions are macular hyperpigmentation with colors ranging from blue-gray to brown. The shape is often irregular and follows the areas of sun exposure, with the face as the most affected area. The use of a Wood's lamp leads to an accentuation of the lesion only in patients with lighter skin types.

Treatment: Lesions evolving from pregnancy may spontaneously disappear following the delivery of a baby and can recur with each subsequent pregnancy. Topical therapy includes hydroquinone (Lustra®, Solaquin Forte®) b.i.d., or 0.1% fluocinolone/4% hydroquinone/0.5% tretinoin (Tri-Luma®) daily at night, plus a sunscreen (containing titanium oxide/zinc oxide) to be worn during the daytime. Some hydroquinone products contain sunscreen or sunblock as well, making it more convenient for the patient to apply. Response usually occurs at 2 months and may take up to 6 months for complete treatment. Patients are advised to continue the use of sunscreen for an additional summer season. Monobenzone (Benoquin®) or other ether compounds of hydroquinone should not be used in melasma because these compounds irreversibly destroy melanocytes, leading to permanent leukoderma.

Chapter **5**

Disorders of Sebaceous and Apocrine Glands

Acne Vulgaris

Acne vulgaris is an inflammatory condition of the pilosebaceous glands with multifactorial causes including genetic disposition, hormones, and the bacteria *Propionibacterium acnes*. These factors interact to cause an increase in sebum production and, subsequently, a breakdown of the lipid in the sebum into fatty acids, which leads to an inflammatory process. Acne is a multifactorial disease that has both physical and psychological effects on patients. The goal for successful treatment of acne is to provide patients with a medication that is effective, well tolerated, and convenient.

Clinical diagnosis: Acne vulgaris commonly occurs on the face and trunk; it may present as comedonal 'whiteheads'/ 'blackheads,' papules, pustules, and nodular cysts.

Treatment: Mild acne (Figure 5-1; see color plate insert) can be treated with topicals, such as benzoyl peroxide (Benoxyl®, Clearasil®, PanOxyl®), or azelaic acid (Azelex®); or topical antibiotic combinations, such as clindamycin/benzoyl peroxide (BenzaClin® b.i.d. or Duac® q.d.); erythromycin/ benzoyl peroxide (Benzamycin® b.i.d.); and clindamycin/ tretinoin (Ziana™ q.d.) for patient convenience (Table 5-1).

For moderate acne (Figure 5-2; see color plate insert), in addition to the topical regimen outlined above, add the following oral antibiotics, listed in order of preference:

Table 5-1: Treatment of Acne Vulgaris

Mild Acne

b.i.d.: Topical antibiotic combinations, such as clindamycin/benzoyl peroxide (BenzaClin®), erythromycin/benzoyl peroxide (Benzamycin®); **q.d.**: clindamycin/benzoyl peroxide (Duac®), clindamycin/tretinoin (Ziana™).

q.h.s.: Topical retinoids, such as tretinoin (Retin-A®) 0.025% cream, 0.05% cream, 0.1% cream; 0.01% gel and 0.025% gel; tazarotene (Tazorac®) 0.05% or 0.1% gel or cream; adapalene (Differin®) 0.1% gel or cream. Topical azelaic acid 20% cream (Azelex®), or 15% gel (Finacea®); topical benzoyl peroxide 2.5%-10% wash (Benoxyl®, PanOxyl®) or benzoyl peroxide 2.5%-10% gel, cream, or wash (Benzac®, Brevoxyl®, Clearasil®, Fostex®, Oxy 10 Balance®, PanOxyl®).

Moderate Acne

In addition to the topical regimen outlined above, add oral antibiotics below:

- First choice: Tetracycline or erythromycin 500 mg b.i.d.
- Second choice: Enteric-coated doxycycline (Doryx®) tablets, 100 mg q.d.
- Third choice: Minocycline (Dynacin®, Minocin®) 50 to 100 mg b.i.d.
- Fourth choice: Trimethoprim/sulfamethoxazole (TMP/SMX) (Bactrim®, Septra®) and clindamycin are used only rarely.

- Tetracycline or erythromycin 500 mg b.i.d. Both of these drugs are listed as first choice only because they are inexpensive. They have no greater efficacy than the other oral antibiotics, but tetracycline has a more difficult compliance because it must be taken on an empty stomach.

Severe Acne

Isotretinoin (Accutane®)

- Usual dose: 0.5 to 1.0 mg/kg/d in two divided doses with food/milk for 15 to 20 weeks.
- Monitoring:
  - Pregnancy: negative test within 1 week of initiation of isotretinoin and then monthly.
  - Two types of birth control from a specific list, 1 month before, during, and posttreatment.
  - Isotretinoin should be started on the second or third day of menstrual cycle.
  - Fasting lipids, complete blood count (CBC), aspartate aminotransferase (AST) at baseline, then monthly.
  - Monitor for possible depression or suicide risk (controversial).

- Doxycycline (Doryx®, enteric-coated capsules), 100 mg q.d. This agent offers once-daily dosing and, unlike minocycline (Dynacin®, Minocin®), does not cause gastrointestinal (GI) or central nervous system (CNS) side effects. As a result, enteric-coated doxycycline capsules tend to have better compliance.

- Minocycline 50 mg to 100 mg b.i.d. This agent has efficacy equal to that of doxycycline enteric-coated capsules but has been associated with GI side effects, such as stomach upset, and CNS side effects, such as dizziness, vertigo, and rarely, lupus-like syndrome.
- Trimethoprim/sulfamethoxazole (Bactrim®, Septra®) and clindamycin are used only rarely.

Severe acne (Figure 5-3; see color plate insert) can be treated with isotretinoin (Accutane®) at a usual dosage of 0.5 mg/kg/d to 1.0 mg/kg/d in two divided doses, taken with food or milk, for 15 to 20 weeks. A second course of therapy can be started after an 8-week period off isotretinoin. Only physicians who are experienced with isotretinoin should prescribe this medication. The following is meant only as a guideline:

Monitoring: Negative serum pregnancy test within 1 week of initiating isotretinoin and then monthly. Fasting lipids, complete blood count (CBC), aspartate aminotransferase (AST) test at baseline, then monthly.

Precautions: Isotretinoin is a category X medication. It should be started on the second or third day of the menstrual cycle. Two types of birth control from a specific list must be taken, 1 month before treatment, during treatment, and 1 month posttreatment. Patient should be monitored for possible depression or suicide risk (controversial).

Rosacea

Rosacea is a chronic inflammatory disorder affecting the blood vessels and pilosebaceous units of the face (Figure 5-4; see color plate insert). Rosacea typically affects the faces of middle-aged adults, occurring more frequently in women than in men. The etiology is unknown.

Clinical diagnosis: Rosacea often has a gradual onset. Usually, the patient first notices erythema; with time, telangiectasia appears. The development of papules and pustules occurs in the later stages. The central forehead, nose, 'butterfly' of cheeks, and the central chin are most

Table 5-2: Treatment for Rosacea

- Topical metronidazole (MetroCream®, MetroGel®) twice daily application
- Oral tetracycline or erythromycin 250 mg to 500 mg twice daily

commonly affected. Rhinophyma, caused by hyperplasia of the sebaceous glands and connective tissue of the nose, sometimes develops in patients with late-stage rosacea, especially if left untreated.

Treatment: Rosacea often requires a combination of topical and systemic treatments (Table 5-2). For mild cases, topical metronidazole, available in both gel (MetroGel®) and cream (MetroCream®) applied twice daily is effective in treating the papules, pustules, and erythema of rosacea. For moderate-to-severe cases, low-dose tetracycline or erythromycin (250 mg to 500 mg, twice daily) is the usual treatment. Most patients respond within 1 month, after which the drug often can be tapered off. If relapse occurs weeks to months later, the antibiotic course can be repeated. If relapse occurs immediately, maintenance on topical metronidazole or reduced daily or every-other-day doses of antibiotic is advised. Systemic isotretinoin is reserved for resistant cases.

Topical steroids are well known to give temporary improvement in appearance by decreasing erythema, but, if used chronically, can cause rebound flare when they are discontinued. Sun exposure can also be an aggravating factor, and sun-protective measures are recommended.

Rosacea is usually chronic, with exacerbations and remissions. Patients usually respond well to therapy. In many, however, therapy must be continued for months to years.

Table 5-3: Treatment for Perioral Dermatitis

- Metronidazole (MetroGel®) 0.75% gel/cream b.i.d.

- Erythromycin 2% gel b.i.d.

- Tetracycline 500 mg b.i.d. until clear, then 500 mg q.d. for 1 month, then 250 mg q.d. for 1 month.

- Doxycycline 100 mg b.i.d. until clear, then 100 mg q.d. for 1 month, then 50 mg q.d. for 1 month.

- Minocycline 100 mg b.i.d. until clear, then 100 mg q.d. for 1 month, then 50 mg q.d. for 1 month.

Perioral Dermatitis

Perioral dermatitis is an idiopathic acneiform inflammatory condition of the perioral and periorbital area, which predominantly affects females of childbearing years.

Clinical diagnosis: Perioral dermatitis has a distinctive distribution with characteristic sparing of vermilion border and the classic physical findings of erythema, papulosis, and scaling.

Treatment: The treatments for perioral dermatitis are listed in Table 5-3. Note that corticosteroids are often not helpful and may exacerbate the condition long term.

Chapter 6

Benign Neoplasms and Hyperplasias

Hypertrophic Scars and Keloids

Keloids and hypertrophic scars are excessive formations of fibrous tissue that develop after cutaneous injuries. Keloids differ from hypertrophic scars in that they extend beyond the original boundaries of injury and often have pseudopod extensions. These lesions can occur at any age with similar prevalence between genders. They occur more often among African Americans.

Clinical diagnosis: Keloids and hypertrophic scars occur after trauma or injury to the site. Lesions are usually papular/nodular and range from flesh-colored to red. Keloids extend beyond the boundary of injury with pseudopod extensions, while hypertrophic scars tend to be more linear. Lesions are often smooth and firm.

Treatment: Intralesional injections of triamcinolone acetonide (Kenalog-10®, Kenalog-40®) 10 mg/mL to 40 mg/mL monthly may reduce the volume of the lesion as well as the pruritus. Lesions that are difficult to inject initially can be treated by liquid nitrogen and allowed to thaw for 15 minutes before injection. Surgical excision is not recommended. Patients who have a history of keloid/ hypertrophic scar formation should be advised against cosmetic procedures such as ear or body piercing.

Skin Tags

Skin tags (acrochordon, cutaneous papilloma, soft fibroma) are benign tumors with a histology of loose fibrous tissue contained within thinned epidermis. They generally occur after middle age and are more prevalent in females and obese patients. Lesions are asymptomatic unless they become irritated because of their location on the body.

Clinical diagnosis: Skin tags are soft peduncles ranging in color from flesh to brown. They are generally located on the neck, eyelids, and intertriginous areas (groin and axilla). Differential diagnosis includes seborrheic keratosis, dermal nevus, neurofibroma, fibroma, and hamartoma.

Treatment: Skin tags are removed through simple snip excision, cryosurgery, or electrodesiccation.

Seborrheic Keratosis

Seborrheic keratosis (SK) is a common benign epithelial tumor. It usually occurs in adults after 30 years of age and is slightly more common in males.

Clinical diagnosis: Lesions initially develop as flesh-colored or brown macules. These lesions later develop into plaques or nodules with a characteristic coarse and 'stuck-on' appearance (Figure 6-1; see color plate insert). Multiple plugged follicles can also occur, as well as a gradual darkening of pigmentation. Lesions may be solitary or generalized and have a predilection to occur on the face, trunk, and upper extremities.

Treatment: Cryosurgery is the simplest way to destroy these lesions, but recurrence is common and histopathologic information is lost. Curettage or shave biopsy with electrocautery of the base may prevent recurrence and allow for definitive histopathologic examination. All suspicious lesions should be sent to dermatopathology to rule out malignancies.

Chapter 7

Diseases Caused by Microbial Agents

Cutaneous Fungal Infections

Cutaneous fungal infections are described with the term 'tinea,' which is an infection of the skin caused by fungal organisms collectively called dermatophytes, followed by a qualifying term denoting the location of the infection on the body (Table 7-1).

Clinical diagnosis: In most dermatophyte infections, the patient presents with a scaling rash. Some of the more common clinical presentations are described in Table 7-1, and include scaling and erythematous, annular (ring-like) plaques and patches, which often have an active, scaly edge and central clearance. Pruritus is common and often the chief complaint of patients.

The most convenient laboratory diagnostic test for dermatophyte infections is the potassium hydroxide (KOH) preparation outlined in Chapter 1. Finding hyphae or pseudohyphae on a KOH preparation is diagnostic of either dermatophytic or candidal infection. Usually, the clinical presentation will distinguish between the two. If necessary, fungal cultures will distinguish between dermatophytic and candidal infections. Cultures are often helpful in cases where dermatophytic infections are suspected, but the KOH examination is negative.

Treatment: Most dermatophyte infections can be adequately treated with topical antifungal agents (Table 7-2). Creams are best for dry areas, while solutions, lotions, or aerosols are best for moist (groin or toe web) or hairy areas

Table 7-1: Cutaneous Fungal Infections

Name	Location	Clinical Appearance
Tinea capitis	Scalp	1. Round, scaling area of alopecia 2. Diffuse scaling 3. Red, boggy, swollen area with pustules (kerion)
Tinea corporis	Body	Annular, 'ringworm'-like, scaly lesions
Tinea cruris	Groin	Sharply demarcated area with elevated, scaling, serpiginous borders
Tinea pedis	Feet	1. Interdigital maceration 2. Diffuse scaling on soles and sides of feet ('moccasin' distribution)
Tinea manuum	Hand	Well-demarcated or diffuse scaling usually on only one palm
Tinea faciale	Face	Slightly scaling, erythematous patches and plaques; border may not be well demarcated in all areas
Tinea unguium	Nails	Thick, brittle, subungual debris with separation of nail plate from the nail bed; commonly show 'dirty yellow' discoloration

Modified from Lookingbill DP, Marks JG Jr: *Principles of Dermatology*. Philadelphia, PA, WB Saunders Co, 1986.

Table 7-2: Topical Antifungal Agents to Treat Cutaneous Candidiasis

Agent	Dermatophytes	Yeast	Tinea Versicolor
Butenafine (Mentax®)	+		
Ciclopirox (Loprox®)	+	+	+
Clotrimazole (Lotrimin® AF, Mycelex®)	+	+	+
Econazole (Spectazole®)	+	+	+
Ketoconazole (Nizoral®)	+	+	+
Miconazole (Femizol®, Micatin®, Monistat-Derm®)	+	+	+
Naftifine (Naftin®)	+		
Nystatin (Mycostatin®)		+	
Oxiconazole (Oxistat®)	+		
Terbinafine (Lamisil®)	+		
Tolnaftate (Tinactin®)	+		+

because they leave little residue and are drying. Powders are poor vehicles for antifungal agents except for use as prophylaxis of interdigital tinea. It is best to treat until a few days after the lesions flatten and stop scaling. Nystatin (Mycostatin®) should not be used to treat dermatophyte infection because it is effective against only *Candida albicans*, a yeast.

Topical corticosteroids can sometimes relieve the itching associated with dermatophyte infection. However, topical corticosteroids can also enhance the cutaneous growth of the fungus, so they should only be used sparingly and short term to control itching.

Systemic therapy is indicated for patients with widespread disease or dermatophyte infections resistant to topical measures. Fungal infection of scalp and nails (finger or toe) also usually requires systemic therapy. The three available systemic antifungal agents are ketoconazole (Nizoral®), itraconazole (Sporanox®), and terbinafine (Lamisil®). Oral ketoconazole is active against systemic fungal infections, *Candida* species, dermatophytes, and deep fungal infections. Side effects occur in <5% of patients; the most common problems are gastrointestinal (GI) upset and pruritus. Transient rises in liver enzyme levels have been observed in some patients, and care should be taken in prescribing oral ketoconazole for patients likely to be at risk of intolerance, including older women, those with a history of liver disease, and those taking other drugs that may affect the liver. Itraconazole is approved in the United States for deep fungal infections in the immunocompromised host and for onychomycosis (fungal infection of the nail bed), but it is also effective against dermatophyte infections and yeast infections. For dermatophyte infections, a dose of 200 mg daily for 1 to 2 weeks is usually adequate. For fingernail infections, a popular regimen is 'pulse dosing,' which consists of a treatment pulse of 200 mg twice daily for 1 week, followed by 3 weeks without itraconazole drug treatment, followed by a second pulse of 200 mg twice daily for 1 week. For toenails, treatment is 200 mg once daily for 12 consecutive weeks. In addition to itraconazole, terbinafine is also effective for the treatment of onychomycosis. The recommended dose is 250 mg ingested daily for 6 weeks for fingernail involvement or 12 weeks for toenail involvement. A common alternative schedule, 'pulse dosing,' is 250 mg taken twice daily for 1 week, repeated once a month for 2 months (fingernails), or 4 months (toenails). The first schedule consumes 84 pills; the second, 56. Unlike ketoconazole and itraconazole, terbinafine has little potential for causing liver disease and does not interact with other drugs using the hepatic P-450 enzyme system, but it occasionally causes GI upset.

Tinea Versicolor

Tinea versicolor is caused by infection with the commensal yeast *Pityrosporum orbiculare*. When the spore forms are transformed to pseudohyphae, infection occurs. Clinically, the lesions appear as finely scaling patches that can be pink, tan, or white, the most common being white ('versicolor' means changing colors). Lesions are most common on the neck, trunk, and upper arms. Occasionally, tinea versicolor is associated with mild pruritus.

Clinical diagnosis: The most useful laboratory diagnostic test is the KOH examination. Examination of the scale with a KOH preparation reveals short, branched pseudohyphae that are often mixed with numerous clustered spores giving an appearance of 'spaghetti and meatballs.'

Treatment: The organism is not contagious and is found in all adults. However, left untreated, it can spread widely and the resulting skin dyspigmentation can be disfiguring. Over-the-counter dandruff shampoo can be used to treat tinea versicolor. It is effective, easy to apply to a widespread area, and relatively inexpensive. This medication can be used in several ways. One is to apply a selenium sulfide shampoo (Exsel®, Selsun®) to the neck, trunk, and upper arms, leave it on for 10 minutes, and then rinse it off. This is done for 3 nights in a row, then weekly for a month, and then once every 3 months to prevent recurrence. Shampoo containing ketoconazole is also effective. Zinc pyrithione shampoos (Head & Shoulders®) have also been successfully used. Topical azole antifungal creams, such as ketoconazole cream, are also effective against the organism, but this approach is expensive when the eruption is widespread, which often occurs.

Oral ketoconazole is a simple and effective therapy. In most adult patients, the fungus may be eradicated with as little as a single 400-mg dose. However, in actual practice, 200 mg ingested twice daily for 5 to 7 days is used to ensure the overgrowth is controlled. Efficacy is enhanced if the patient works up a sweat 2 hours after ingesting the medication, thereby enhancing delivery of the drug, which is concentrated in sweat, to the stratum corneum. For patients with recurrent disease, this regimen can be repeated every 3 months for 1 year.

Treatment clears scaling quickly, but color may not return to normal for 2 to 3 months. Recurrences are common. After topical therapy, the recurrence rate is >50%, but can be reduced to <15% with the every-3-month retreatment program described above. It is important to explain this to the patient so that on recurrence, he or she will not view the treatment as a failure.

Cutaneous Candidiasis

Candidiasis (candidosis, moniliasis) is a superficial yeast infection caused by *Candida* species (*C albicans* is the most common). These infections can occur at any age, and there is no difference in prevalence between genders. Infections generally occur only when predisposing factors are present, such as occlusion, heat, moisture, and altered immunity (ie, diabetes, HIV infection). Patients with occupations that involve frequent contact with water (ie, health-care workers, hair stylists, florists) may also be at risk. Classifying candidiasis by anatomic location may help determine treatment regimens.

Clinical diagnosis: Physical examination varies by anatomic location. Potassium hydroxide preparations of scrapings show pseudohyphae and budding yeast. Although fungal cultures may aid in identification of *Candida* species and bacterial cultures may aid in ruling out superinfections, neither is necessary to establish the diagnosis.

Cutaneous candidiasis categories include:

Intertrigo—is a nonspecific inflammation of body folds, such as axillae, inframammary, groin, and gluteal folds, which may be caused by *Candida* infections. Early infections appear as pustules on an erythematous base that later evolve into sharply demarcated erythematous, eroded patches. Discrete small pustular lesions (satellite lesions) occur near the primary lesion and are pathognomonic for candidiasis.

Occluded skin regions—such as areas under occlusive dressing and diapers, under casts, and on the backs of hospitalized patients—present with a clinical picture similar to intertrigo.

Erosio interdigitalis blastomycetica—another form of candidiasis, occurs in web spaces of fingers and toes. The lesion appears as an oval-shaped area of macerated white skin on the web space. As the condition progresses, the macerated skin peels, leaving a painful, raw, denuded area surrounded by a collaret of scales.

Genital candidiasis—presents as balanitis in males and vulvovaginitis in females. Physical examination reveals pustules, erythema, erosions, and white plaques.

Oropharyngeal candidiasis (thrush, *Candida* leukoplakia)—primarily occurs in patients who are immunocompromised (ie, diabetes, HIV, transplant recipient), who are debilitated, or who use inhaled/systemic corticosteroids. Infections present as white plaques on the buccal mucosa, hard/soft palate, pharynx, and tongue, which, when removed, may cause bleeding on the mucosal surface. Ody-

Table 7-3: Treatment for Candidal Vulvovaginitis

- Clotrimazole (Gyne-Lotrimin®, Mycelex®):
  1% cream, 1 full applicator q.h.s. x 7 d
  100-mg tablet intravaginal q.h.s. x 7 d
  200-mg tablet intravaginal q.h.s. x 3 d
  500-mg tablet intravaginal q.h.s. x 1 d

- Miconazole (Femizol®, Monistat®):
  2% cream, 1 full applicator q.h.s. x 7 d
  100-mg tablet intravaginal q.h.s. x 7 d
  200-mg tablet intravaginal q.h.s. x 3 d
  1200-mg tablet intravaginal q.h.s. x 1 d

- Fluconazole (Diflucan®):
  150 mg PO single dose

nophagia (pain with swallowing) is a marker for invasive esophageal *Candida* infection and should be a cause for concern; these patients should be referred to a gastroenterologist for diagnosis and treatment.

Treatment: Common treatments for cutaneous candidiasis are listed in Table 7-2. Treatments for candidal vulvovaginitis are listed in Table 7-3.

For oropharyngeal *Candida* infections, clotrimazole oral trouche (10 mg) PO, 5 times/day may be effective. Immunocompromised patients may need daily *Candida* infection prophylaxis with either oral fluconazole or ketoconazole.

Folliculitis

Folliculitis is the infection and inflammation of hair follicles. The types of infection include bacterial (ie, *Staphy-*

lococcus aureus, Pseudomonas aeruginosa, other gram-negative bacteria), viral (herpes simplex virus [HSV]), and fungal (ie, dermatophytes, *Candida*). Predisposing factors include shaving, hair extraction (waxing), use of contaminated hot tubs, skin occlusion (skin folds or external dressings, such as plastic wrap/bed sheets), topical corticosteroid use, hot humid climate, immunocompromised state (ie, diabetes, HIV, organ transplant recipients), and alteration of natural skin flora (certain oral antibiotics). Folliculitis can evolve into furuncles (abscess formation) and carbuncles (contiguous furuncles).

Clinical diagnosis: Clinical history provides important clues to causative organisms. Most folliculitis is caused by *S aureus,* while 'hot tub' folliculitis is caused by *P aeruginosa.* An immunocompromised state may lead to nonbacterial and bacterial infections. Folliculitis is characterized by erythematous papules and pustules located at the base of the hair follicle with surrounding erythema (Figure 7-1; see color plate insert). Extensive folliculitis may appear as confluent erythematous plaques with erosions and crusting. Laboratory tests, such as hematoxylin and eosin (H&E) staining of the skin biopsy specimen to visualize bacteria, fungus, or virus (viropathic changes in the cells), as well as bacterial and fungal cultures of the biopsy specimen may aid in distinguishing the different forms of folliculitis if empiric therapy fails.

Treatment: Treatment is dependent upon the causative organisms. Most folliculitis and mild furuncles respond to local warm compresses (to aid spontaneous drainage) and cleansing with antibacterial soap or benzoyl peroxide. If conservative treatment is ineffective, apply topical mupirocin ointment (Bactroban®) twice a day to the affected area for 2 weeks and nares for 5 days to reduce nasal carriage of *S aureus*. First-choice oral antibiotics include cephalexin (Keflex®) or dicloxacillin, both 250 mg to 500 mg q.i.d. for 10 days (although chronic folliculitis may require months of antibiotic therapy). Alternative second-choice oral an-

Table 7-4: Treatment of Folliculitis

Folliculitis and Mild Furuncles

- Local warm compresses (to aid spontaneous drainage)

- Antibacterial soap

- Benzoyl peroxide

- Topical mupirocin ointment (Bactroban®) b.i.d. to the affected area for 2 weeks and to the nares for 5 days to reduce nasal carriage of *S aureus.*

Resistant Folliculitis (in order of preference)

- Cephalexin (Keflex®) or dicloxacillin, both 250 mg to 500 mg q.i.d. for 10 days (although chronic folliculitis may require months of antibiotic therapy)

- Erythromycin, first- or second-generation cephalosporins (with adequate gram-positive coverage), clindamycin, or amoxicillin/ clavulanate (Augmentin®)

tibiotics include erythromycin, first- or second-generation cephalosporins (with adequate gram-positive coverage), clindamycin, and amoxicillin/clavulanate (Augmentin®). 'Hot tub' folliculitis is usually self-limited, and antibiotics are not necessary. For carbuncles and furuncles with signs of surrounding cellulitis (with or without fever), oral antibiotics and drainage are indicated (Table 7-4).

Lice and Scabies
Head Lice

Head lice (*Pediculus humanus capitis*) infest the scalp and can cause an extremely pruritic condition. Infestations are more common in children, but can occur in all ages. Head lice are transmitted by sharing hats, brushes, or bedding, and through physical contact.

Clinical diagnosis: Diagnosis is confirmed by seeing the lice and/or nits. Head lice are six-legged, wingless insects approximately 1 mm to 4 mm in size. They are often difficult to detect on the scalp because the average lice population per patient is fewer than 10. Diagnosis is often made through the discovery of nits, oval white eggs of head lice averaging 0.5 mm in size, which can number in the thousands. Nits adhere to the hair shaft as hair emerges from the follicle. Nits are found near the scalp during recent infestations and further down the hair shaft after longer infestations. With scratching and excoriations, some areas may also be secondarily infected. Although head lice infest scalp hair, infestation of eyelashes is also seen.

Pubic Lice

Pubic lice (crabs, crab lice) are infestation by *Phthirus pubis*. Areas of involvement include the pubic area as well as other hairy parts of the body, such as the axillae, chest, and eyelashes. Since pubic lice live on humans and do not usually wander, transmission is caused by close physical contact or possibly by sharing towels.

Clinical diagnosis: Diagnosis is confirmed by the presence of the lice and/or nits. Pubic lice are six-legged, wingless insects around 1 mm to 2 mm in size; the mouth is usually embedded in the skin with the claws grasping a hair on either side.

Treatment: In treating head lice or pubic lice (Table 7-5), the surrounding environment must be thoroughly vacuumed. All head gear, clothing, and bedding require washing and drying on the hot cycle. Combs and brushes should be soaked in alcohol or other disinfectants for 1 hour. Sex partners must also be treated. Avoiding contact with contaminated items is the best prevention.

Table 7-5: Treatment for Lice

- Permethrin, 5% prescription strength (Elimite®) cream

- Permethrin, 1% nonprescription strength (Nix®) lotion/cream rinse

The preferred drug treatment regimen includes permethrin, 5% prescription strength (Elimite®) cream, or permethrin, 1% nonprescription strength (Nix®) lotion/cream rinse. Wash hair with a medicated shampoo for 10 minutes, then rinse off. It is extremely important to use a special fine-tooth nit comb to remove the nits. Enzymatic lice egg removers (Clear® shampoo) are also available over the counter. Since the incubation period for lice eggs is 6 to 10 days, the entire process should be repeated in 7 to 14 days.

Scabies

Scabies is an infestation by the mite *Sarcoptes scabiei*. Although transmission usually occurs through close physical contact, mites can live outside of the human body for up to 2 days, so physical contact is not absolutely necessary. Scabies infestation in an otherwise healthy person generally results in a small mite population (ie, <10); however, patients who are immunocompromised or who suffer from neurologic disorders are at risk for crusted (ie, Norwegian) scabies, in which the mite population can occur in the millions.

Pruritus in scabies is caused by a hypersensitive reaction to the mite. Therefore, in unexposed patients, pruritus may develop several weeks after the initial infestation and subsequent sensitization. In previously exposed patients, pruritus may develop within 1 day. The pruritus associated with scabies may be intense and generalized with the exception of the head and neck. Although most patients experience pruritus, 50% of patients with crusted scabies do not experience pruritus.

Clinical diagnosis: Intraepidermal burrows are almost pathognomonic for scabies. Burrows are a few millimeters long with linear or serpiginous ridges, and appear as superficial, short, thin, delicate white lines. Each burrow is produced by a single female mite and may extend to 10 cm in length during prolonged infestation. There may be a tiny papule or vesicle at the end where the female resides and lays eggs. Burrows are usually found in nonhair-growing regions with thin stratum corneum (ie, fingers, web spaces, wrists, elbows). Infestations can also occur on the head and neck in infants. Pruritic inflammatory nodules in the scrotum of male patients often signify scabies infection.

Mites can be seen in the KOH or oil prep of thin superficial skin from the affected area. The burrow is superficially sliced off with a scalpel, usually without anesthetic. The extremely thin specimen is placed on a slide with a few drops of KOH or mineral oil, and covered with a coverslip. Mites, eggs, and mite feces may all be seen in the preparation.

Cutaneous manifestations of hypersensitivity reaction, such as urticaria and eczematous dermatitis, can occur in scabies infestation. Long-standing infestation can also produce stigmatas of chronic pruritus, such as excoriations, lichen simplex chronicus, and prurigo nodularis. Areas of infestation may also have secondary infections that require additional treatment.

Treatment: Avoiding contact with contaminated items is the best prevention. When an infestation occurs, the surrounding environment should be thoroughly vacuumed and all clothing and bedding washed and dried on the hot cycle, or removed from the body for a minimum of 72 hours. Sexual partners and anyone with personal

Table 7-6: Treatment for Scabies

**Immunocompetent Patient
(in order of preference)**

- Permethrin 5% cream

- Sulfur 6% to 10% in petrolatum q.d.
  for 3 days and repeated in 1 week

- Ivermectin* (Stromectol®) 200 µg/kg PO once

Immunocompromised Patient

Complete eradication may be impossible,
so multiple treatments are advised.

- Day 1: Permethrin as above

- Days 2 to 7: Sulfur 6% to 10% in petrolatum q.d.,
  which should be repeated for several weeks.

*Investigational for this condition

or household contact within the preceding month should
be examined and treated, if necessary. Pruritus is controlled with antihistamines and topical corticosteroids.
Severe hypersensitivity reaction may be treated with a
prednisone taper of 1 to 2 weeks. Pruritus may persist for
several weeks after treatment because of the continued
hypersensitivity to dead mites.

The treatment regimen for an immunocompetent patient
(in order of preference) includes permethrin 5% cream,
sulfur 6% to 10% in petrolatum once daily for 3 days and
repeated in 1 week, and ivermectin (Stromectol®) 200 µg/kg
PO once (Table 7-6).

Apply permethrin 5% cream from head to toes and leave
on for 8 to 10 hours. Repeat in 1 week. Fingernails should
be trimmed, and permethrin should be reapplied after

handwashing. This regimen is not recommended during pregnancy, but is safe for children older than 2 months.

Complete eradication of scabies may not be possible in immunocompromised patients, and multiple treatments are advised.

- Day 1: Permethrin as above.
- Days 2 to 7: Sulfur 6% to 10% in petrolatum once daily, which should be repeated for several weeks.

Molluscum Contagiosum

Molluscum contagiosum (MC) is caused by two subtypes of the molluscum contagiosum virus, MCV-1 and MCV-2, which belong to the poxvirus family. Infections occur via skin contact in children and sexual activity in adults; HIV patients are at risk for multiple facial mollusca.

Clinical diagnosis: Molluscum contagiosum presents as small, flesh-colored, round papules or nodules with central umbilication. The area of distribution includes exposed skin in children, genital areas in adults, and facial areas in HIV patients. Resolving lesions are often surrounded by erythema.

Treatment: Molluscum contagiosum in normal hosts usually resolves spontaneously within 6 months. In HIV patients, the condition may progress despite therapy. Current therapy includes curettage, cryosurgery, and electrosurgery.

Herpes Zoster

Herpes zoster ('shingles') is caused by the reactivation of latent varicella-zoster virus (VZV) after primary varicella infection (chicken pox). The incidence is highest in the elderly and in conditions such as AIDS, Hodgkin's disease, lymphoma, and immunosuppressive therapy. It is characterized by groups of vesicles on an erythematous base in a dermatomal distribution. A prodrome of radicular pain and itching often precedes the eruption. The eruption may affect more than one dermatome. Bilateral involvement is rare.

Table 7-7: Treatment for Herpes Zoster

- Oral acyclovir (Zovirax®)
  800 mg 5 x daily for 7 to 10 days
- Oral famciclovir (Famvir®)
  500 mg 3 x daily for 7 days
- Oral valacyclovir (Valtrex®)
  1 g 3 x daily for 7 days
- Appropriate analgesics

Clinical diagnosis: The dermatomal distribution of herpes zoster is diagnostic. It can be confirmed by a Tzanck preparation, direct immunofluorescence (DIF) staining of vesicle smear, or viral culture in the few cases where the diagnosis is uncertain.

When herpes zoster involves the tip of the nose, suspect eye involvement because the nasociliary branch of the ophthalmic division of the trigeminal nerve innervates the eye and the tip of the nose. Zoster of the ophthalmic division of the trigeminal nerve may lead to corneal ulcers and scarring.

Treatment: Mild attacks; may only need rest, analgesics, and bland applications, such as calamine lotion. When the vesiculopustules of herpes zoster rupture, crusting and weeping are reduced with acetic acid astringent compresses.

Oral acyclovir (Zovirax®) should be used for symptomatic cases at a dose of 800 mg 5 times daily for 7 to 10 days. Famciclovir (Famvir®) and valacyclovir (Valtrex®) are alternatives to acyclovir (Table 7-7). Treatment is most effective when started within the first 3 days of an attack. For immunocompromised patients, disseminated zoster, and ophthalmic zoster, intravenous acyclovir should be used at a dose of 10 mg/kg every 8 hours.

A potential complication from herpes zoster is postherpetic neuralgia, which occurs most commonly in the elderly. Amitriptyline at a dose of 25 mg to 50 mg daily or capsaicin analgesic cream 0.025%-0.075% (Zostrix®, Zostrix®-HP) used topically 3 or 4 times daily on affected skin can provide pain relief. Postherpetic neuralgia becomes asymptomatic in 12 months for 80% of patients.

Herpes Simplex Virus: Oral and Genital Infections

Herpes simplex is a viral infection caused by HSV. Grouped vesicles on an erythematous base are characteristic of HSV infection. The vesicles quickly become pustules, which rupture, weep, and crust. Herpes simplex virus has been separated into two types—HSV-1 and HSV-2. Usually HSV-1 causes oral infection, and HSV-2 causes genital infection. However, either type can infect any area of skin.

Herpes simplex virus is transmitted by skin-to-skin contact. Primary infection with HSV-1 usually occurs in children. In 90% of cases, the infection is subclinical, while the remaining 10% develop acute gingivostomatitis. Primary infection with HSV-2 is usually transmitted sexually and causes multiple, painful genital or perianal blisters, which rapidly ulcerate. Primary infections are frequently accompanied by systemic symptoms including fever, malaise, myalgias, headache, and regional adenopathy. Primary herpes infection persists for about 3 weeks.

Fifty percent of patients will have recurrent attacks at certain characteristic sites after varying periods of latency, during which the virus remains dormant within the dorsal root ganglion corresponding to the site of the infection. Recurrences may be precipitated by a number of factors, including fever, ultraviolet light, physical trauma, menstruation, or emotional stress. Tingling, burning, or even pain is followed within a few hours by the development of erythema and clusters of tense vesicles. Crusting occurs

Table 7-8: Recommended Dosages of Acyclovir for Herpes Simplex

	Immunocompetent Patient
First-episode genital herpes	400 mg 3 times daily for 7 to 10 days
Recurrent genital herpes	400 mg 3 times daily for 5 days
Herpes prophylaxis	400 mg twice daily for up to 12 months

within 24 to 48 hours. Recurrent episodes have a shorter course of 1 to 2 weeks.

Clinical diagnosis: A history of a vesicular eruption recurring in the same general location should lead to a suspicion of HSV infection. The diagnosis of herpes simplex is made clinically. If necessary, it can be confirmed with a Tzanck smear, DIF, or viral culture.

Treatment: Acyclovir is the drug of choice for HSV infections. It selectively inhibits viral DNA polymerase and replication of viral DNA. It is effective against replicating virus, but does not eliminate latent virus. If administered promptly, acyclovir decreases healing time, viral shedding, and duration of symptoms.

Acyclovir is available in topical and systemic preparations. Acyclovir ointment 5% is effective only for primary HSV infection. Topical acyclovir has little clinical benefit in active recurrent infection. Oral acyclovir is effective against primary and recurrent HSV infections. Intravenous acyclovir is indicated in the treatment of severe primary HSV

Immunosuppressed Patient

400 mg 3 times daily orally for 7 to 14 days, or 5 to 10 mg/kg every 8 hours intravenously for 7 to 14 days. May add topical acyclovir 4 to 6 times daily.

400 mg 3 times daily orally for 7 to 14 days, or 5 to 10 mg/kg every 8 hours intravenously for 7 to 14 days. May add topical acyclovir 4 to 6 times daily.

400 mg 3 times daily orally (lower or higher according to response).

and initial and recurrent infections in immunocompromised patients. Treatment does not prevent recurrent infection. Oral acyclovir prophylaxis is recommended for patients who experience 6 or more attacks per year. Recommended acyclovir dosages are presented in Table 7-8. Famciclovir and valacyclovir dosages are listed in Table 7-9.

Immunocompromised patients are most at risk for developing complications from HSV infections. These complications include chronic ulcerative herpes simplex, which lasts for weeks to months; generalized acute mucocutaneous herpes simplex; and systemic infection involving the liver, lungs, adrenals, and central nervous system (CNS).

Human Papillomavirus Infections
Cutaneous Nongenital Warts

Warts are caused by various subtypes of human papillomaviruses (HPV). The three most prevalent types are common warts (*verruca vulgaris*), plantar warts (*verruca plantaris*), and flat warts (*verruca plana*). Transmission

Table 7-9: Recommended Dosages of Famciclovir and Valacyclovir for Herpes Simplex

	Famciclovir	Valacyclovir
First-episode genital herpes	250 mg 3 times daily for 7 to 10 days	1,000 mg twice daily for 7 to 10 days
Recurrent genital herpes	1 g twice daily for 1 day	500 mg twice daily for 3 days
Recurrent herpes labialis	1.5 g single dose	2 g twice a day for 1 day; separate doses by 12 hours
Herpes prophylaxis	250 mg twice daily for up to 1 year	500 mg to 1,000 mg once daily for up to 1 year
Recurrent oral/ genital herpes in HIV patients	500 mg twice daily for 7 days	1 g twice daily for 5 to 10 days
Herpes prophylaxis in HIV patients	500 mg twice daily	500 mg twice daily

occurs via skin contact and is facilitated by cutaneous trauma; however, laser and electrosurgery may also result in airborne transmissions. Immunocompromised patients and meat handlers are at increased risk.

Clinical diagnosis: Common warts present as small hyperkeratotic firm papules that are flesh colored. When superficial layers are shaved off with a scalpel, they may reveal red or brown dots, which are thrombosed

Table 7-10: Treatment for Cutaneous Nongenital Warts

- May resolve spontaneously within months to a few years
- Salicylic acid or lactic acid in collodion solutions applied q.d.
- 40% salicylic acid plaster (Mediplast®) before using solutions for large lesions
- Cryosurgery
- Electrosurgery

capillaries. This simple procedure is useful in making a distinction between warts and calluses, the latter having a semitransparent nucleus instead of thrombosed capillaries upon shaving.

Plantar warts usually present near the pressure points of the foot as small, sharply demarcated papules/plaques with hyperkeratotic surfaces. Because of their locations, plantar warts may be painful. Thrombosed capillaries and complete disruption of dermatographics distinguishes plantar warts from corns (keratoses) and calluses. Flat warts present as a group of sharply demarcated flat papules (1 mm to 2 mm in elevation). Papules may be linear (as the result of trauma) and confluent.

Treatment: Cutaneous nongenital warts generally resolve spontaneously within months to a few years; therefore, treatment may not be warranted and may lead to scarring. Daily application of over-the-counter salicylic acid/lactic acid/collodion for up to 12 weeks to small lesions cure 70% to 80% of cases. Larger lesions (primarily palmar or plantar warts) may require a 40% salicylic acid plaster (Mediplast®) to be applied before the use of solutions. The salicylic acid plaster should first be cut to size, then secured in place with strong skin tape. The plaster should be changed every 24 hours following filing with a nail file. Cryosurgery involves freezing the wart with a 1-mm to 2-mm margin as frequently as every 4 weeks until complete resolution. Large warts may require curettage to debulk the lesion before cryosurgery. Electrosurgery may be more effective than cryosurgery, but may also increase the chance of scarring (Table 7-10).

Anogenital Warts

Anogenital warts (*condylomata acuminata*, acuminate/venereal warts, *verruca acuminata*, mucosal warts) are caused by various subtypes of HPV in the anogenital region. Transmission occurs via sexual and nonsexual skin contact, and is facilitated by cutaneous trauma. Laser surgery and electrosurgery may also result in airborne transmissions. Genital warts in children may be a marker for sexual abuse, although anogenital warts can also be acquired through vaginal deliveries. Children who aspirate viral particles during vaginal deliveries are at risk of developing respiratory papillomatosis. Finally, certain subtypes of HPV infections are now believed to cause anogenital dysplasia and carcinoma, such as cervical cancer; therefore, women with genital warts should be encouraged to have annual Pap smears as a part of cervical cancer screening. Patients with genital warts should also be screened for other sexually transmitted diseases, including HIV.

Clinical diagnosis: Anogenital warts range in appearance from flesh-colored papules to large, exophytic masses, distributed in mucosal and adjacent areas. Although they are almost always found in clusters, genital warts may also be found singly. Subclinical mucosal infections may not be visible until 5% acetic acid is applied for a period of time to turn the involved surface whiter than the surrounding skin (aceto-white test).

Table 7-11: Treatment for Anogenital Warts

- Prevention through use of barrier contraceptives
- Cryosurgery (weekly or biweekly)
- Trichloroacetic acid (up to 80% to 90%) may be applied to warts weekly, for up to 6 weeks
- Imiquimod 5% cream (Aldara™) applied 3 times/wk at bedtime and washed off in 6 to 10 hours
- Podophyllum resin and its standardized extract podofilox (Condylox®)
- Electrosurgery
- Laser surgery

Treatment: The best treatment for anogenital warts is prevention through the use of barrier contraceptives. There is currently no cure for genital warts, only symptomatic treatments. In some cases, untreated lesions spontaneously resolve after several months. Despite aggressive treatments, recurrence is common and generally represents reactivation of subclinical infections rather than reinfections from sexual partners. Imiquimod 5% cream (Aldara™) applied 3 times/wk at bedtime and washed off in 6 to 10 hours for up to 16 weeks is a useful first-line treatment that can be used at home. Cryosurgery, performed weekly or biweekly, is safe and rarely results in scarring. Trichloroacetic acid (up to 80% to 90%) may be applied to warts weekly for up to 6 weeks. Podophyllum resin and its standardized extract, podofilox (Condylox®), can be used to treat genital warts. Podophyllum resins (up to 25% concentration) are applied focally by physicians to warts and washed off after 1 to 4 hours. Sessions are repeated weekly for up to 6 weeks. Podofilox 0.5% solution can be used for self-treatment and is applied by cotton swab twice daily for 3 days, followed by 4 days without treatment (up to 4 cycles). Because of systemic absorption, the total area treated by podophyllum or podofilox must be <10 cm^2 and the total volume of medications used must be <0.5 mL/day. Both podophyllum and podofilox are teratogenic and are contraindicated during pregnancy. Finally, electrosurgery and laser surgery are highly effective and may be used if other therapies fail (Table 7-11).

Syphilis

Syphilis is a sexually transmitted disease caused by *Treponema pallidum*. After a 10- to 90-day incubation period, the primary lesion appears as a painless ulcer (chancre) at the site of inoculation. Untreated, it lasts about 6 weeks and is usually accompanied by local lymphadenopathy.

Secondary syphilis starts 4 to 12 weeks after the appearance of the primary chancre. The chancre is usually (but not always) healed by the time the secondary phase develops, but the patient may recall it. The secondary phase of syphilis represents an inflammatory response in the skin and mucous membranes to the hematogenously disseminated *T pallidum*. The rash of secondary syphilis can mimic many other skin disorders. The most common lesions are 'ham-colored' scaling papules and plaques. The eruption is often generalized and classically involves the palms and soles. Systemic symptoms are usually present, including fever, headache, myalgia, arthralgia, sore throat, and malaise. A general guideline to remember is that for patients with a generalized rash of unknown origin accompanied by systemic complaints, a test for secondary syphilis should be administered.

Clinical diagnosis: The diagnosis of syphilis can be ruled out by a nonspecific serologic test for syphilis, rapid plasma reagin (RPR). A positive RPR should be confirmed by a fluorescent treponemal antibody absorption (FTA-ABS) test, which is a more specific test for syphilis. Positivity of these two blood tests confirms the diagnosis. The serologic test for syphilis may be negative in a patient with coexisting HIV infection and secondary syphilis. If syphilis is suspected in this setting, a darkfield examination and/or biopsy of a skin lesion can confirm the diagnosis. These procedures visualize the spirochetes in serous fluid obtained from the lesion or in special stains of biopsy material. Patients diagnosed with syphilis should also be tested for HIV infection because the presence of the former is a risk factor for acquiring the latter.

Treatment: Penicillin remains the treatment of choice for syphilis. For primary and secondary syphilis in immunocompetent patients, a single intramuscular injection of benzathine penicillin (Bicillin® L-A) 2.4 million units is adequate therapy. Erythromycin or tetracycline 500 mg 4 times daily for 15 days, or doxycycline 100 mg twice daily for 14 days, are effective alternatives for immunocompetent patients who are allergic to penicillin. HIV-infected patients require more intensive therapy, either with weekly benzathine penicillin injections for 3 weeks or with a course of intravenous aqueous penicillin or intramuscular ceftriaxone (Rocephin®). With therapy, many patients experience a febrile reaction (Jarisch-Herxheimer reaction) typically beginning within 12 hours and resolving within 1 day.

Secondary syphilis is highly contagious. Without therapy, the lesions of secondary syphilis spontaneously resolve in 1 to 3 months in immunocompetent patients. With therapy, the lesions resolve promptly. The FTA-ABS test often remains positive indefinitely.

In the secondary phase, the treponemal organism spreads not only to the skin but also to other organs. Hepatitis occurs in approximately 10% of patients, bone and joint disease in approximately 4%, and nephritis even less often.

Approximately one third of untreated patients develop complications of syphilis (tertiary syphilis) years later, of which the most important are cardiovascular and CNS manifestations. In patients with HIV infection, progression to tertiary syphilis is more frequent and can occur within months after primary infection.

Chapter **8**

Miscellaneous Dermatologic Disorders

Lichen Planus

Lichen planus (LP) is an idiopathic inflammatory condition that involves the skin, its associated structures, and mucous membranes. It commonly affects patients between 30 and 60 years of age, with no predilection for either gender. Current evidence suggests that autoimmune factors are involved in its pathogenesis, although this theory has yet to be substantiated. Many medications are known to cause LP-like lesions that resemble the idiopathic condition both clinically and histologically. Oropharyngeal involvement is associated with a higher incidence of oropharyngeal carcinoma.

Clinical diagnosis: Lichen planus characteristically presents as pruritic, violaceous (bluish-purple), flat-topped papules and plaques with sharply defined edges. The surface is shiny and often has a white, lacy pattern (Wickham's striae). Lesions are usually found symmetrically on the flexural surfaces of wrists and forearms, sides of the neck, thighs, shins, lower back, and genital region. Mucous membrane involvement, ranging from the oropharynx (especially buccal mucosa) to the urogenital area, presents in about 60% of cases and manifests as lacy, reticulated (net-like), white striae on the mucosa. Scalp lesions may present as follicular papules associated with scarring alopecia, and nails may develop longitudinal grooving and splitting (pterygium).

Variations on the characteristic papules, descriptions of which are beyond the scope of this text, include hypertrophic, bullous, follicular, erosive, atrophic, actinic, and malignant degenerations. Biopsy often confirms the diagnosis.

Treatment:

Discrete lesions
- Topical corticosteroids
- Intralesional corticosteroid injections (triamcinolone acetonide [Kenalog-10®, Kenalog-40®])

Oral lesions
- Corticosteroids (topical, lozenges, aerosol, pellets)
- Topical anesthetics (Orabase®)
- Cyclosporine mouthwash

Recalcitrant/widespread lesions
- Oral corticosteroids (short course with rapid taper)
- Cyclosporine (Neoral®) at 3 to 5 mg/kg q.d. (divided into b.i.d. dosing to minimize side effects)
- Retinoids (ie, acitretin [Soriatane®]) at 30 mg/day.
- Psoralen/ultraviolet light A (PUVA) phototherapy

Both topical pimecrolimus (Elidel®) and tacrolimus (Protopic®) have been used successfully in the treatment of LP when steroid resistance or side effects are encountered.

Drug Eruptions

Fixed Drug Eruption

Fixed drug eruption (FDE) is a drug hypersensitivity reaction in which the same area of skin is involved each time the patient is systemically exposed to a certain chemical. An idiopathic process, FDE occurs within hours of exposure. Oral medications are the most common offending agents, but food and food additives have also been implicated.

Clinical diagnosis: A history of an identical lesion occurring at the same site following exposure to certain foods or drugs is indicative of FDE. Some patients may mistakenly associate certain events, rather than the triggering agent, with the lesions (eg, headaches or colds rather than cold medications). Fixed drug eruption usually presents as

Table 8-1: Treatment of Fixed Drug Eruption (FDE)

- Withdrawal of offending agent
- Topical corticosteroids

a single erythematous macule/patch, which may progress to a plaque, bulla, and finally, to an erosive ulcer. Although mostly solitary, FDE may also present as multiple lesions and mimic other cutaneous disorders, such as Stevens-Johnson syndrome (SJS). Most lesions occur in the genital region, but all other mucocutaneous areas may be susceptible.

Treatment: Fixed drug eruption is treated by identification and withdrawal of the offending agent. In patch or plaque stages, FDE may be treated with topical corticosteroids. Ulcerated areas should be covered with antibacterial ointments such as bacitracin (Neosporin®) or mupirocin (Bactroban®, Centany™) and covered until reepithelization is complete (Table 8-1).

Exanthematous Drug Eruption

Exanthematous drug eruption (EDE) is the most common type of drug hypersensitivity reaction, characterized by a maculopapular rash that occurs following exposure to a drug. Although it rarely has systemic involvement, EDE may also be the initial presentation of a more serious adverse hypersensitivity condition, such as SJS.

Clinical diagnosis: During initial sensitization, an eruption can occur anytime from the first day to 3 weeks after exposure to the drug, with a peak incidence at 9 days. In a previously sensitized person, the eruption usually occurs 2 to 3 days after exposure. Interestingly, almost all patients with Epstein-Barr virus (EBV) or cytomegalovirus (CMV) infections will develop this condition after administration

Table 8-2: Treatment of Exanthematous Drug Eruption (EDE)

- Identification and withdrawal of offending agent.

- Patient may have cross-reactivity to other medications and should be warned.

- Oral antihistamines may be given to control pruritus.

- Topical corticosteroid may help speed the resolution of eruption.

- Oral or intravenous corticosteroids are generally not indicated unless the offending drug must be continued.

of penicillin or amoxicillin. The patients are pruritic and may have a fever. The rash resembles a viral exanthem in which multiple erythematous macules and/or papules often become confluent especially in intertriginous areas. Lesions are usually symmetric and almost always occur on the trunk and extremities.

Treatment: To treat EDE, identify and withdraw the offending agent. The patient may have cross-reactivity to other medications and should be advised on prevention. Oral antihistamines may be given to control pruritus, and topical corticosteroids may help speed the resolution of an eruption. Oral or intravenous corticosteroids are generally not indicated unless the offending drug must be continued (Table 8-2).

Typically, it will take 2 weeks for the rash to resolve. Patients with fever or eosinophilia should have a full work-up to rule out systemic involvement (drug rash with eosinophilia and systemic symptoms [DRESS] syndrome) in which the liver and the kidneys are often affected. If elevated, liver function test (LFT) and creatinine test should be followed.

Stevens-Johnson Syndrome and Toxic Epidermal Necrolysis

Stevens-Johnson syndrome and toxic epidermal necrolysis (TEN) are life-threatening mucocutaneous conditions that require acute hospitalization. Both SJS and TEN are considered part of the same process, with TEN at the severe end of the disease spectrum with more generalized involvement. The conditions may be idiopathic, but in many cases, they are drug induced. The incidence in both genders is the same.

Clinical diagnosis: Obtaining the patient's history of new drug use is important in diagnosing SJS and TEN; exposure to any new drug within the past 3 weeks must be suspected. There may be a prodrome of malaise and fever several days before presentation. Tenderness and diffuse erythema of the skin and mucosa often exist that may at first resemble an EDE. There may be bullous formation with positive Nikolsky's sign (lateral spread with pressure applied gently to the top of the blister). The skin in TEN is characteristically tender to the touch. The clinical picture quickly evolves over several days to extensive full-thickness epidermal detachment revealing exposed dermis. Topical epidermal necrolysis is associated with significant mortality. If the patient survives, regrowth of epidermis follows after several more days and is usually completed within 3 weeks.

Treatment: Acute hospitalization and monitoring in a burn unit or an intensive care unit is required since SJS and TEN are life-threatening. The mortality rate associated with SJS is <5%, and approximately 30% for TEN. The use of intravenous hydration and electrolyte management are important because of the substantial loss of epidermis. Corticosteroids are unlikely to be effective. Associated morbidity from bacterial superinfection is high, and any signs of infection should be treated aggressively.

Table 8-3: Drugs That Commonly Cause Photosensitivity

- Amiodarone (Cordarone®, Pacerone®)
- Chlorpropamide (Diabinese®)
- Nalidixic acid (NegGram®)
- Oral contraceptives
- Phenothiazines
- Psoralens
- Quinidine
- Sulfonamides
- Tetracycline, doxycycline (Doryx®, Vibramycin®)
- Thiazides

Photodermatitis

Phototoxic Reaction

Clinical diagnosis: There are drugs that may absorb ultraviolet radiation and cause phototoxic drug reactions. Some drugs that can cause phototoxic reactions are listed in Table 8-3. Most of these drugs absorb ultraviolet light A (UVA) as well as ultraviolet light B (UVB) radiation. As a result, window glass, which is protective against the UVB rays primarily responsible for sunburn, will not protect against most phototoxic drug reactions. Phototoxic reactions are not immunologic. Every person who is exposed to enough of the triggering drug and to enough ultraviolet radiation will develop a phototoxic reaction.

Phototoxic reactions present as a sunburn. Redness and tenderness occur on exposed areas, such as the backs of hands and arms, the 'V' area of the upper chest, sides, and back of the neck, the nose, the chin, the forehead, and the ears. The

Table 8-4: Features That Distinguish Phototoxicity From Photoallergy

Phototoxicity	Photoallergy
Erythematous reaction	Eczematous reaction
Immediate reaction	Delayed reaction
Pain	Itchiness
Negative photopatch test	Positive photopatch test

condition usually spares the eyelids, the area under the brows, the upper lip under the nose, and the submental region.

Treatment: Treatment of a phototoxic reaction is the same as for a sunburn. The drug should be discontinued, and the patient protected from additional ultraviolet light exposure (avoidance, clothing, and sunscreens with UVB and UVA blocking effects).

Photoallergic Reaction

Clinical diagnosis: Many of the same drugs that cause phototoxic reactions can also cause photoallergic reactions. Ultraviolet radiation converts an immunologically inactive form of a drug into an antigenic molecule. An immunologic reaction analogous to allergic contact dermatitis occurs on subsequent exposure to the drug and ultraviolet radiation. The primary differences between phototoxicity and photoallergy are detailed in Table 8-4.

The original lesions are red patches, plaques, vesicles, or bullae, which usually become eczematous. The areas exposed to ultraviolet radiation become inflamed, but the reaction is more likely to be eczematous. The eruption will be on exposed areas such as the hands, the 'V' area of the neck, the nose, the chin, and the forehead. There is also a tendency to spare the upper lip under the nose, the eyelids, the submental region, and behind the ears. Often, the eruption does not occur on the first exposure to ultraviolet light, but only after the second or further exposures. A lag phase of 1 week or more is necessary to induce an immune response.

Photopatch testing can confirm the diagnosis. The chemical is applied for 24 hours, and the skin is then irradiated with UVA, eliciting an acute photoallergic contact dermatitis. A control patch, which is not irradiated, rules out ordinary (ie, nonphotoinduced) allergic contact dermatitis.

Treatment: A photoallergic reaction tends to resolve when either the drug or the exposure to ultraviolet radiation is stopped, but this may take several weeks. Use of a potent topical corticosteroid or a short course of systemic corticosteroid hastens resolution and provides symptomatic relief.

Urticaria and Angioedema

Urticaria is the result of dermal edema, while angioedema is the result of subcutaneous edema. The two may occur either simultaneously or separately. Etiology and testing for each condition is detailed in Table 8-5.

Clinical diagnosis: History is important. Urticarial wheals are transient, pink areas of dermal edema, sometimes surrounded by an erythematous halo (Figure 8-1; see color plate insert). Generally round or oval, they may also be linear in the case of dermatographism (urticaria caused by stroking of the skin). Urticaria is generally pruritic, and the wheals usually spontaneously resolve after 12 hours. Discrete urticarial wheals that last >24 hours should raise suspicion for a systemic diagnosis, such as urticarial vasculitis. Angioedema manifests as well-demarcated subcutaneous edema with a predilection for the eyelids, lips, tongue, larynx, and gastrointestinal (GI) tract.

Treatment: Prevention of attacks is important, especially when the etiologic agent has been identified (ie, food, inhalant, drugs). Antihistamines are the mainstay of treatment. Doxepin (Sinequan®), a tricyclic antidepressant, has powerful H_1 and H_2 blocking properties and is the treatment choice if diphenhydramine (Benadryl®) and hydroxyzine are ineffective. The initial dose of doxepin is 25 mg/night, and may be titrated upward by 25 mg/wk, up to the usual effective adult dose of approximately 100 mg/night. The maximum dose is 300 mg, based on clinical response and tolerance. Since doxepin can cause conduction abnormalities (QT prolongation), a screening electrocardiogram should be performed to document a normal QT interval and the absence of cardiac arrhythmias in patients who are older than 55 years or who have a history of cardiac conduction abnormalities. Systemic glucocorticoids as a long-term therapy are generally avoided in idiopathic, allergen-induced, and physical urticarias; however, they are useful in pressure/vibratory urticaria, urticarial vasculitis, and idiopathic angioedema. In addition, hereditary angioedema in male patients can be treated with danazol, an attenuated androgen, while pediatric and female patients may be treated with aminocaproic acid (Amicar®), an antifibrinolytic agent.

Drug-Induced Urticaria and Angioedema

Drug-induced urticaria and angioedema is a drug hypersensitivity reaction in which urticaria and/or angioedema occurs after exposure to an offending drug. Because this condition may herald anaphylaxis (which can include respiratory compromise and shock), the patient must be carefully observed.

Immune Mediated

- Immunoglobulin E (IgE) mediated: Drug recognized by host IgE, which in turn triggers mast cell degranulation, leading to urticaria and angioedema. Occurs at 7 to 14 days after initial sensitization, but further exposures tend to result in immediate reactions (eg, antibiotics).

Table 8-5: Etiology and Testing for Urticaria and Angioedema

Type	Etiology/Features
Acute urticaria (<6 weeks)	
• IgE mediated	
Food/inhalant	1. Frequently patient has atopic diathesis.
	2. Food additives (benzoic acid and azo dyes) can cause chronic urticaria.
Parasite	Eosinophilia
• Complement mediated	Mast cell degranulation caused by complement activation (ie, serum sickness).
• Drug induced	See section on drug eruptions.
Chronic urticaria (>6 weeks)	
• Idiopathic urticaria	80% to 90% of chronic urticaria
• Physical urticaria	
Dermatographic	Affects 4% to 5% of the general population.
Cold urticaria	Located at sites of contact with cold surfaces.
Solar urticaria	Characteristic light exposure distribution.
Cholinergic urticaria	Small (<5 mm) micropapular wheals.

IgE = immunoglobulin E

Diagnostic Test

Antigen challenge (food/inhalant)

Skin patch testing or radioallergosorbent test (RAST)

Stool for ova and parasites x 3
By history only

N/A

Light stroking of the skin incites wheal
and flare reaction.
Ice cube or test tube of ice water x 10 minutes.
Wheal develops within 5 minutes of removal.

UVA, UVB, visible light x 30 to 120 seconds on a
small test location. Wheal develops within 30 minutes.
Exercise or hot shower to the point of perspiration
causes micropapular wheals.

(continued on next page)

Table 8-5: Etiology and Testing for Urticaria and Angioedema *(continued)*

Type	Etiology/Features
• Physical urticaria *(continued)*	
Pressure/vibratory urticaria	1. No laboratory abnormalities 2. Vibration may cause direct mast cell degranulation. 3. Large, painful, red swellings at pressure sites (soles, palms, wrists)
Urticaria vasculitis	1. Discrete wheals lasting >24 hours. 2. May have concomitant purpura.
Hereditary angioedema	Autosomal dominant

• Complement mediated: Drug recognized by antibodies, resulting in the formation of immune complexes and activation of the complement system, leading to the release of anaphylatoxins and mast cell degranulation. Occurs at 7 to 10 days, but can occur up to 1 month after initial exposure (eg, serum sickness).

Nonimmune Mediated

• Direct mast cell degranulation: Drug causes direct mast cell degranulation without antibody intermediaries (eg, radiographic contrast media, polymyxin B, curare, *d*-tubocurarine).

Diagnostic Test

Pressure/vibratory stimulus

Biopsy of wheal at the edge should include portions of the wheal as well as the normal dermis.

Low C4 levels
Low levels or dysfunctional C1 esterase inhibitor

- Disruption of arachidonic acid metabolism: Drugs that block the cyclooxygenase pathway and inhibit prostaglandin synthesis. Occurs 30 minutes to 4 hours after exposure (eg, aspirin-induced asthma, nonsteroidal anti-inflammatory drugs [NSAIDs]-induced rhinitis).
- Disruption of kinin metabolism: Angiotensin-converting enzyme (ACE) inhibitors block kinin metabolism, which is believed to be the cause of ACE inhibitor-associated angioedema (0.1% to 0.2% incidence). Patients undergoing hemodialysis are at higher risk (up to 35%).

Table 8-6: Treatment of Urticaria and Angioedema

- Identify and withdraw the offending agent.

- Antihistamines, but doxepin (Sinequan®), a tricyclic antidepressant that has powerful H_1 and H_2 blocking properties, is the choice of treatment if diphenhydramine (Benadryl®) is ineffective.

- Respiratory distress will require protection of airway.

- Epinephrine (0.3 mg to 0.5 mg of a 1:1,000 dilution) SQ every 15 minutes for bronchospasm.

- Systemic corticosteroids (IV or oral) may be necessary for severe cases.

Clinical diagnosis: The patient's history of drug exposure is critical. Physical examination shows urticaria and angioedema (see section on urticaria/angioedema for more details).

Treatment: Table 8-6 outlines treatment options for urticaria and angioedema.

Cysts

Epidermoid Cyst

Epidermoid cysts (wen, sebaceous cyst, infundibular cyst) are the most common type of cyst. They are derived from the epidermis or the epithelium of a hair follicle, forming a lined cavity within the dermis. The epidermoid cyst contains keratin and lipids. As long as the cyst remains intact, there is no inflammation and the cyst remains asymptomatic. However, cysts often rupture into the surrounding dermis because of their thin epithelial lining, creating an inflammatory response.

Clinical diagnosis: An epidermoid cyst presents as a mobile dermal or subcutaneous nodule, often with a central pore. The cyst is usually located on the face, neck, or upper trunk. If ruptured, the content of the cyst is a creamy paste-like material with a rancid odor. Rupture of the cystic material into the surrounding dermis may provoke an inflammatory response, causing erythema, tenderness, and what looks like an infection.

Treatment: A ruptured and inflamed cyst may require intralesional injection of a corticosteroid to control the inflammation, possibly followed by surgical removal once the inflammation is completely resolved. The injection does not have to be within the sac, since it has ruptured and the content is already in the surrounding tissue. An antibiotic (eg, erythromycin, 500 mg twice daily) may be helpful for its anti-inflammatory effect and its bactericidal effect if a secondary infection is present.

Pilar Cyst

Pilar cyst (trichilemmomal cyst, isthmus catagen cyst) is usually found in the scalp and is the second most common type of cyst. It is derived from epidermal cells, forming a lined cavity within the dermis; unlike the epidermoid cyst, the epithelial lining in the pilar cyst is usually thick. Pilar cysts are often familial, occurring more often in females.

Clinical diagnosis: A pilar cyst presents as a mobile dermal or subcutaneous nodule without a central pore. Most are located on the scalp, and the overlying hair is normal. Rupture of the content may also cause an inflammatory reaction; however, a pilar cyst is usually more solid than the epidermal inclusion cyst and, therefore, much less likely to rupture.

Treatment: Pilar cysts are removed via surgical excision, which removes the entire epithelial lining.

Chapter **9**

Precancerous Skin Lesions and Skin Cancer

Actinic Keratosis

Actinic keratosis, also called solar keratosis, is a premalignant condition that can sometimes progress to squamous cell carcinoma. It is caused by sun damage to exposed areas of patients with skin types 1 to 4 on the skin-type scale (type 1 is the most easily sunburned and type 6 is the least). Actinic keratosis occurs mostly in middle-aged or older people, with a higher prevalence in males. People with higher geographic, occupational, or recreational sun exposures are at greater risk.

Clinical diagnosis: Actinic keratosis presents as small, scaly, pink or brown papules. A rough, gritty (sandpaper-like) consistency on palpation often aids in diagnosis. Often, actinic keratoses are easier to appreciate on palpation than on visual inspection. Lesions may be solitary or in groups, and occur on sun-exposed areas of the body.

Treatment: Cryosurgery with liquid nitrogen is the treatment of choice for actinic keratosis and is applied with adequate duration to obtain an approximately 1-mm margin around the lesion over 2 cycles; patients are examined in 1 month and remaining lesions undergo another round of cryosurgery. Extensive lesions can be treated twice a day with 5% 5-fluorouracil cream (Efudex®) for 2 weeks, or once a day with 0.5% 5-fluorouracil cream (Carac®) for up to 4 weeks or twice a day for 2-6 weeks with 1% 5-fluoro-

Table 9-1: Treatment of Actinic Keratosis

- Cryosurgery with liquid nitrogen
- 5-fluorouracil cream
  (Carac® [0.5%], Efudex® [5%], Fluoroplex® [1%])
- Diclofenac (Solaraze®) gel
- Imiquimod (Aldara™) cream

uracil cream (Fluoroplex®) (Table 9-1). Treatment is also effective using 3% diclofenac gel (Solaraze®) twice daily for 3 months. Finally, 5% imiquimod cream (Aldara™) used twice weekly for 16 weeks or 3 times weekly for 4 weeks is also effective in the treatment of extensive actinic keratosis. Patients should be warned to expect intense erythema, ulceration, and crusting at the treatment area, possibly 5 to 15 days after initiation of therapy. It is believed that the inflammation achieved may aid in the clearance of actinic keratosis. Cessation of the medication and symptomatic relief will allow the areas to heal completely. If necessary, topical corticosteroids can be used in combination to reduce the intensity of the reaction.

Dysplastic Nevus

Dysplastic nevi (also called *atypical moles*) were previously considered to be markers for increased risk of melanoma in family members with a rare, familial form of melanoma, the familial atypical mole and melanoma syndrome or dysplastic nevus syndrome. In these families, virtually all members with atypical moles developed a melanoma at some point, while family members without atypical moles did not. Subsequently, it was discovered that approximately 5% of the normal white population in the United States has atypical moles. The risk of these people developing a melanoma, many of whom have only one or a few atypical moles and

Table 9-2: Guidelines for Follow-Up of Patients With Dysplastic Nevi

Baseline Evaluation:

- Shave biopsy of at least two most clinically atypical lesions to confirm diagnosis.

- Total skin photographs, including closeups of suspicious lesions.

Follow-up Frequency:

- Patients with no personal or family history of melanoma: every 12 months.

- Patients with personal or family history of melanoma, every 3 months for 2 years. If no changes, then every 6 months for 3 years. Then periodically reevaluate at the discretion of the physician.

Modified from Lookingbill DP, Marks JG Jr: *Principles of Dermatology.* Philadelphia, PA, WB Saunders Co, 1986.

no personal or family history of melanoma, is unclear, but most of them will never develop a melanoma.

Moles are either congenital or acquired. Most moles are acquired after 6 months of age and before 35 years of age. There is a more rapid development of moles during adolescence, and a slower development during the first half of adult life. It is common to have darkening in color, itching, and development of new nevi during pregnancy and adolescence.

Clinical diagnosis: The most important task is to differentiate a benign mole from a dysplastic nevus and melanoma. Moles vary greatly in appearance and color. They can be flat or elevated, smooth or verrucous, polypoid or sessile, and pigmented or flesh-colored. Uniform color, uniform surface, and sharply demarcated and regular borders are characteristic features of a benign mole that differentiate it from a dysplastic nevus or melanoma. A dysplastic nevus is usually >5 mm, is variegated in color, and has an irregular border. In addition, nevi that have recently changed in color, shape, or size, and symptomatic nevi (eg, those that itch or bleed spontaneously) should be regarded as suspicious. If there is any doubt, a biopsy should be performed.

Treatment: A shave biopsy is recommended if a lesion is suspected of being a dysplastic nevus. However, if melanoma is suspected, a full-thickness biopsy is necessary for diagnosis and prognosis. Individuals with multiple atypical moles but no personal or family history of melanoma should be educated about sun exposure, self-skin examination, and have yearly or more frequent full-skin examinations by a physician. Guidelines for patient follow-up are outlined in Table 9-2.

Skin Cancer

Skin cancer is the most common type of cancer: 1 in 5 whites will develop skin cancer during their lifetime. Sun exposure appears to be the primary cause of skin cancer. Sun damage that occurs in childhood and young adulthood is the most important factor in determining future skin cancers. It is estimated that 80% of the total lifetime sun exposure occurs in the first 18 years of life. Invisible skin damage builds up over many years, and skin cancer can result.

Basal Cell Carcinoma

Basal cell carcinoma (BCC) is the most common type of skin cancer, comprising approximately 80% of total cases. It affects about 800,000 people annually in the United States. Most BCCs occur in sun-exposed skin in fair-skinned people, particularly in the head and neck areas.

Clinical diagnosis: Classically, BCC consists of a pearly (translucent), flesh-colored papule or nodule that often has a depressed center or crater, a rolled border, and telangiectasia. It can sometimes be superficial and

Table 9-3: Treatment for Basal Cell Carcinoma (BCC)

- Surgical excision
- Curettage and electrodesiccation
- Cryotherapy
- Radiation therapy
- Mohs' chemosurgery

appear as a shiny, thin patch or plaque, and rarely, it can also be pigmented.

The diagnosis of BCC should be confirmed through either a shave or punch biopsy. The techniques of skin biopsy are reviewed in Chapter 1. Patients with BCC should be considered for a referral to a dermatologist for treatment.

Treatment: Destructive treatments of BCC have a cure rate of >95% in uncomplicated cases. Each method (Table 9-3) has advantages and disadvantages. Tumor site, type, patient age, and cosmetic needs all help determine the method that is right for each patient. The most frequently used forms of therapy are surgical excision and curettage and electrodesiccation. Surgical excision is generally preferred if the lesion is small, simple, and easily closed. The procedure is usually quick and involves minimal postoperative inconvenience. The cosmetic outcome is good and, most importantly, the margins of the surgical specimen can be checked for adequacy of excision.

Curettage and electrodesiccation is an effective treatment for simple, superficial lesions, and possibly for those with a larger diameter. An unsightly scab is present for weeks, and residual scarring is usually marked but may be slight on certain areas of the face. The adequacy of treatment is detected by the 'feel' of the curettage in the hands of an experienced dermatologist; BCCs are much softer than normal dermis. The surgical specimen is fragmented and useless for determining margins. Curettage and desiccation should be performed only by adequately trained clinicians.

Cryotherapy consists of tissue destruction via repeated cycles of freezing and thawing with liquid nitrogen spray or metal applicators. A generous margin is selected clinically to ensure adequate treatment. Pain, swelling, tissue necrosis, and oozing may last for days to weeks after therapy. Often, there is surprisingly little scarring. Cryotherapy tends to spare cartilage, so it may be useful for treating tumors on the nose and ear. It should be performed only by an experienced dermatologist. Radiation therapy is appropriate for complex tumors but is particularly harmful to cartilage. It requires 10 to 20 office visits and is followed by weeks of inflammation. Radiation is usually reserved for elderly patients who desire a nonsurgical approach. The scar has a good early appearance, but may look worse with the passage of years and may undergo malignant degeneration, generally restricting the use of this modality to patients more than 60 years of age. Lastly, superficial subtypes of BCC may be treated topically by 5% 5-fluorouracil (Efudex®) cream twice daily for 3 to 9 weeks or by 5% imiquimod (Aldara™) cream 5 times weekly for 6 weeks. Although topical treatments may lead to ulceration or erosions, the cosmetic outcome is generally good. Because treatment of superficial BCC with topical therapy involves the ability to recognize clearance of tumor, these modalities should only be used by experienced physicians.

Recurrent tumors have a cure rate of only 50% when treated by curettage, cryotherapy, or radiation therapy. Surgical excision with examination of the specimen for clear margins is the best treatment. For difficult primary or recurrent tumors, the preferred treatment is often Mohs' chemosurgery, or microscopically controlled serial excisions. The tumor is mapped and excised, and the margins are immediately checked on frozen sections. Areas abutting positive margins are immediately excised and checked, and this continues until all specimens are clear. With this technique, the cure rate for primary and recurrent tumors is >95%.

Basal cell carcinomas rarely metastasize but may enlarge locally and can invade underlying tissues, resulting in significant morbidity and mutilation. Follow-up examinations should be performed at 3, 6, and 12 months, and yearly or twice yearly thereafter, because approximately 35% of patients will develop another BCC within 5 years.

Squamous Cell Carcinoma

Squamous cell carcinoma (SCC) is a malignant tumor of keratinocytes (skin and mucous membranes). The incidence of SCC in the United States is 80,000 to 100,000 cases annually, with incidence in males almost twice that in females. Although the major predisposing risk factor for SCC is fair skin (skin phototypes 1 and 2), numerous environmental carcinogens play a role in its pathogenesis. Exogenous carcinogens now believed to cause SCC include arsenic, hydrocarbons, thermal radiation, solar radiation, roentgen radiation, topical nitrogen mustards, systemic or topical psoralen/ultraviolet light A (PUVA) therapy, scarring, and human papillomavirus, in particular HPV-16, -18, -31, -33, -35, and -45. Immunosuppression, such as in transplant patients, may also predispose a person to the development of SCC.

As with other types of oncogenesis, SCC probably develops through a multistep process. The current disease model is that SCC arises from precancerous lesions, progressing to in situ SCC, and finally transforming into invasive SCC.

The classification of SCC is listed in Table 9-4.

Clinical diagnosis: In situ SCC refers to full-thickness intraepidermal SCC. Once the SCC transverses the basement membrane and extends into the dermis, it is referred to as invasive SCC. Carcinoma must be ruled out by biopsy in any slowly growing keratotic or eroded papule that persists for more than 1 month.

Table 9-4: Classification of Squamous Cell Carcinoma (SCC)

Precancerous Lesions

- Actinic keratosis
- Arsenic keratosis
- Tar keratosis
- Radiation keratosis

In Situ SCC

- Bowen's disease
- Erythroplasia of Queyrat

Invasive SCC

- Highly differentiated SCC
- Poorly differentiated SCC

Bowen's disease is a single lesion most commonly seen as an enlarging erythematous plaque with a discrete border. There may be some crusting and scaling, similar to a psoriatic lesion. Although this lesion usually occurs in sun-exposed skin, Bowen's disease can occur in all areas exposed to environmental carcinogens. Erythroplasia of Queyrat specifically refers to Bowen's disease that occurs on the penis or the vulva. The histology and pathology of the two are identical.

Invasive SCCs are usually small, firm, flesh-colored or erythematous nodules. They can be classified as highly or poorly differentiated based on their histopathology (Table 9-4). Highly differentiated SCCs show keratinization and hence, are firmer on palpation than a poorly differentiated SCC, which does not show keratinization.

Treatment: Squamous cell carcinoma is treated through surgical excision. Cutaneous SCC in the sun-exposed area of the anatomy has a low incidence of metastasis. Although the overall metastasis rate is 3% to 4%, SCC arising from nonactinic keratosis may have a rate of metastasis as high as 20% to 30%. Overall remission rates may be as high as 90%, with SCC from actinic keratosis having the highest rate.

Melanoma

Melanoma is a malignant neoplasm of pigment-forming cells, melanocytes, and nevus cells. Excluding other skin cancers, melanoma accounts for 2% of all cancers and 1% of all cancer deaths in the United States.

While the exact pathogenesis of melanoma is unknown, certain risk factors exist for developing melanoma (Table 9-5). Simply being fair-skinned is a risk for melanoma. Melanoma is rare in blacks and Asians, most often found on the palms and soles of the foot or affecting the mucous membranes. In whites, the leg is the most common site in women, and the back is the most common site in men. Only 30% of melanomas arise from moles; the remainder arise from normally pigmented skin.

Clinical diagnosis: Early diagnosis is the key to improving the prognosis in this potentially fatal disease. Clinically, its hallmarks are an irregularly shaped and deeply pigmented papule or plaque. It is important to remember the ABCD of melanoma (Table 9-6). An increase in mole size or change in color is noted in at least 70% of the patients who have melanoma. Development of a new growth, bleeding, and itching are other symptoms that may accompany a melanoma.

There are three clinical types of melanoma, which differ considerably in appearance, behavior, and prognosis (Table 9-7). Lentigo maligna melanoma appears as a slow-growing, dark macule typically on the face of an elderly white person. It has an irregular border and indistinct edges, with various shades of brown, tan, and black hyperpigmentation. It may be present for many years as a macule (malignant cells confined to the epidermis), but may eventually develop

Table 9-5: Risk Factors for Melanoma

- Skin type 1 or 2
- Blonde or red hair
- Light-colored eyes (green, blue, or gray)
- Excessive sun exposure during childhood and teen years
- Blistering sunburns before the age of 20
- Family history of melanoma or atypical moles
- More than 100 moles on the body
- More than 50 moles if under age 20

an invasive nodule (lentigo maligna melanoma) and may metastasize in the nodular stage. It is less aggressive than the other two types.

Superficial spreading melanoma appears as a slightly elevated plaque anywhere on the body. It has an irregular border with areas of blurring of pigment into surrounding skin in various shades of black, brown, and white. It may have a rim of pink inflammation. The surface is slightly fragile and may bleed or ooze. It grows as a small plaque (cells in epidermis and upper dermis) for 6 to 24 months and then develops a nodule, which is highly invasive. There is a >90% cure rate with complete excision in the plaque stage, but prognosis is poor after the nodule develops.

Nodular melanoma arises suddenly as a papule or nodule on the skin or in a mole (Figure 9-1; see color plate insert). It is a blue-black or brown nodule that bleeds easily, often with a rim of inflammation. It is occasionally flesh-colored. Metastasis can occur in only weeks or months (cells spread rapidly into dermis and blood vessels). Occasionally, nodular melanoma will involute after metas-

Table 9-6: Melanoma Signs (ABCD)

- **A**symmetry—a mole that is not the same on both sides

- **B**order irregularity—scalloped or poorly demarcated border, 'coast of Maine' type of border

- **C**olor variability within the same lesion—black, brown, gray

- **D**iameter— >0.5 cm or the size of a pencil eraser

tasis (10% of patients with metastatic melanoma have no remaining primary lesion). Prognosis is poor without early and complete excision.

Any patient who has an abnormal mole or is concerned should probably be referred to a dermatologist. Experience in evaluating lesions is critical. It is imperative that all suspicious pigmented lesions be biopsied. If melanoma is suspected, a full-thickness biopsy, rather than a shave biopsy, must be performed because it is crucial to be able to determine the thickness of the lesion. Prognosis is related to tumor thickness. Generally, the prognosis is excellent for patients with shallow lesions (<0.75 mm) and worsens in proportion to their depth. Performing partial biopsy of a melanoma and reexcising the remainder later does not increase the incidence of metastasis. If the histology confirms the diagnosis of melanoma, physicians should refer the patient to a center experienced in melanoma treatment as soon as possible.

Treatment: Surgical excision is recommended for all melanomas. Follow-up examinations for lentigo maligna or thin superficial spreading melanoma should be performed at 6 and 12 months after excision and yearly thereafter. Thicker nodular lesions are followed up at 6-month intervals with physical examination for metastases. Metastatic

Table 9-7: Three Clinical Types of Melanoma

Type	Approximate Percentage of Cases
Lentigo maligna	10
Superficial spreading melanoma	70
Nodular melanoma	20

melanomas usually respond poorly to radiation therapy and chemotherapy, and prognosis is poor. These patients should be referred to an oncology center.

Cutaneous T-Cell Lymphoma

Cutaneous T-cell lymphoma (CTCL), also known as mycosis fungoides, is a malignancy of helper T-cells (CD4+) with primary cutaneous manifestations. In advanced stages, the disease may progress to extracutaneous manifestations, such as involvement of internal organs. Cutaneous T-cell lymphoma presumably evolves from precancerous lesions; however, these premalignant conditions are exceedingly difficult to diagnose, with histologic findings showing mature lymphocytes and nonspecific inflammation. In fact, eczema and psoriasis are the two most commonly diagnosed conditions before a definitive diagnosis of CTCL, illustrating the nonspecific inflammatory characteristics of the premalignant condition. Thus, premalignant conditions are often diagnosed in retrospect, with a latent period between onset and a definitive diagnosis of CTCL of approximately 4 to 10 years.

Clinical diagnosis: Because of the difficulty in establishing a definitive diagnosis of CTCL, any patients with dermatoses that are recalcitrant to conventional treatment should be considered for biopsies at periodic intervals to rule out CTCL.

Cutaneous T-cell lymphoma can present at different morphologic stages: patch, plaque, tumor, and erythrodermic. Patch stage is characterized by single or multiple erythematous, scaly macules and patches that are well defined and vary in size. Because phototherapy is a treatment for CTCL, these lesions tend to occur in unexposed areas of the body. Lesions may be pruritic or nonpruritic, and may regress spontaneously.

Plaque stage CTCL may arise from patch stage CTCL or may develop de novo. The CTCL plaques are elevated, scaly, well demarcated, and vary in color from red to violaceous.

Tumor stage CTCL may arise from patch/plaque stage or may develop de novo. Tumors have an affinity for the face and skin folds, although they can be found anywhere on the body. It is believed that the evolution from patch or plaque stages to tumor stage reflects the development of vertical growth in the malignancy, while a de novo occurrence suggests metastases. The tumors present as firm nodules that are occasionally ulcerated and may be secondarily infected.

The erythrodermic stage (Sézary syndrome) can develop from the other stages of CTCL or develop de novo. This stage is characterized by diffuse erythema and scaling of the skin, which may resemble erythroderma of other conditions such as psoriasis, atopic dermatitis, generalized contact dermatitis, and drug eruptions.

Treatment: While a detailed explanation of these modalities is beyond the scope of this book, treatments for CTCL include topical chemotherapy, radiotherapy, PUVA, and chemotherapy.

Chapter 10

Common Hair Disorders

Hair loss problems can be divided into two categories—scarring alopecias, which are associated with permanent injury to the hair follicle, and nonscarring alopecias, which are associated with changes in the hair cycle. The three most common hair loss disorders are the nonscarring alopecias—androgenetic alopecia, telogen effluvium, and alopecia areata. Characteristics of these disorders are detailed in Table 10-1.

When evaluating a patient who presents with hair loss, it is important to take a thorough history, physical examination, and in some cases, laboratory tests and biopsy. Important elements of the history include the age of onset, pattern of hair loss, course of hair loss (acute vs gradual), associated scalp symptoms (itching, burning, tingling), medications taken, recent emotional or physical stress, diet, hair-care habits, and family history of baldness or hair disorders. For women, it is also important to inquire about menstrual cycle and reproductive history.

Important elements of the physical examination include the pattern of hair loss (patterned, patchy, diffuse), the areas affected (scalp vs eyebrows/eyelashes vs whole body), and whether scarring is present. Patchy hair loss is readily apparent. However, diffuse hair loss may not be noticeable until there is more than 50% hair loss. The presence or absence of scarring is important diagnostically and prognostically. In nonscarring alopecia, the diagnosis is usually made without biopsy. In scarring alopecia, a

Table 10-1: Common Hair Disorders

Factor	Androgenetic Alopecia
Hair loss distribution	Patterned hair loss
Course	Gradual onset with progression
Appearance	Thinning, with or without bare patches
Shedding	Minimal
Age at onset	Puberty or older
Pull test	Usually negative

Modified from Hordinsky MK, Sawaya ME, Scher RK: *Atlas of Hair and Nails.* Philadelphia, PA, WB Saunders Co, 2000.

biopsy is useful in establishing the diagnosis and should be performed. Nonscarring alopecia may be a temporary phenomenon, whereas scarring is indicative of permanent hair loss. In addition, it is important to look for other signs of androgen excess in the female patient, such as acne vulgaris or hirsutism.

Androgenetic Alopecia

Androgenetic alopecia (male or female pattern baldness) represents postpubertal replacement of the coarse, dark terminal hairs by finer, depigmented (vellus) hairs in areas of baldness, and eventually, completely atrophic follicles. It occurs in genetically predisposed males and females. There is usually a family history of baldness.

The onset and progression of androgenetic alopecia are gradual. Baldness characteristically occurs in a distinctive

Telogen Effluvium	Alopecia Areata
Generalized	Usually patchy, but can be generalized
Abrupt onset, trigger factor	Abrupt onset, often waxes and wanes with relapses
Thinning with no bare patches	Thinning with abrupt bare patches
Prominent	Prominent
Any age	Any age
Positive, resting (telogen) hairs in early stage	Positive, resting hairs primarily

pattern that spares the posterior and lateral margins of the scalp. In men, the process begins with bitemporal recession, followed by balding of the vertex. In women, androgenetic alopecia most often begins with diffuse thinning of the entire top of the scalp. In areas of baldness, the scalp appears completely normal with no evidence of scarring or inflammation.

Clinical diagnosis: The diagnosis is usually straight-forward in men. In women, the diagnosis of androgenetic alopecia may be more difficult. Hormonal abnormality should be considered in women with baldness, particularly if accompanied by acne and/or hirsutism. Women should be asked about menstrual irregularities and infertility, but for most, androgenetic alopecia is simply an inherited trait.

Treatment: Minoxidil (Rogaine®) solution applied topically twice daily can be an effective treatment for androgen-

Table 10-2: Treatment Options for Androgenetic Alopecia

- Hair pieces
- Hair enhancers (shampoos, mousse products)
- Electromagnetic fiber particles (to hide scalp color in light-skinned people)
- Topical minoxidil (Rogaine®) twice daily
- Oral finasteride (Propecia®) 1 mg once daily
- Hair transplantation

etic alopecia. It stops or reduces the rate of hair loss and restores lost hair in some patients. After 1 year of treatment, approximately 30% of men and a slightly higher percentage of women achieve moderate-to-dense regrowth of terminal hairs. Younger men with thinning hair (but not completely bald) respond best. This treatment is also effective in older women with thinning hair. The vertex of the scalp is the most responsive; the frontal region is the least.

Oral finasteride (Propecia®) 1 mg once daily is another treatment option for men with androgenetic alopecia. Finasteride blocks the enzyme 5α-reductase type II, preventing the conversion of testosterone to dihydrotestosterone (DHT). In the adult male, DHT is associated with alopecia, acne, and prostate enlargement. Dihydrotestosterone is important in the normal development of a male fetus because an adequate DHT level is required to develop normal male genitalia. It is not understood what role DHT plays later in life.

Androgenetic alopecia is slow to respond to treatment with either minoxidil or finasteride. It can take months before there is a noticeable change in hair growth, so users should be encouraged to be patient. In addition, new hair growth is not permanent; it reverses when treatment is stopped. Current recommendations for both minoxidil and finasteride are to continue therapy to maintain results. Hair regrowth generally plateaus after about 1 year and may slowly decline over subsequent years. Extensive areas of baldness can be covered with a hairpiece or wig. For selected patients, surgical treatment with hair transplantation or scalp reduction is successful. A summary of treatment options can be found in Table 10-2.

Telogen Effluvium

Marked emotional or physiologic stress may result in an alteration of the normal hair cycle and in the diffuse but potentially reversible hair loss known as telogen effluvium. The scalp is composed of a mosaic of growing (anagen) and resting (telogen) hairs. Telogen effluvium, or stress-induced alopecia, is characterized by excessive and premature entry of growing anagen hairs into the resting telogen phase. The number of resting telogen hairs is increased from a normal percentage of 10% to 20% to >25%, which results in as many as 400 to 500 hairs lost daily. Normally, fewer than 100 hairs are lost daily. The mechanism for this alteration of the normal hair cycle is unknown.

Clinical diagnosis: Telogen effluvium occurs most often in postpartum women. Patients often characterize their hair loss as hair coming out by 'handfuls' after combing and shampooing. Other causes of telogen effluvium include high fever, severe illness, major surgery, severe emotional disorder, crash dieting, and drugs (eg, heparin, warfarin, boric acid, indomethacin, nitrofurantoin, sulfasalazine, thyroxine, vitamin A, anticancer drugs). However, it is not always possible to elicit the cause of the hair loss from the patient.

Upon physical examination, there is diffuse thinning of the hair that may not be readily apparent to the examiner. The scalp is normal, with no scarring or erythema. In telogen effluvium, gentle pulling of the hair (hair-pull test) verifies excessive hair shedding, performed by grasping a group of 2 dozen to 3 dozen hairs and applying gentle traction. Normally, fewer than 3 hairs are pulled out. Pulling out more than 5 hairs confirms that excessive shedding is present.

Patient history and physical examination are usually diagnostic of telogen effluvium. Metabolic causes of diffuse, nonscarring alopecia must be differentiated from telogen effluvium. Abnormal thyroid function, particularly hypothyroidism, can produce diffuse hair shedding, often with loss of the lateral third of each eyebrow. Nutritional deficiencies (eg, lack of an essential fatty acid, biotin, or zinc) or anemia can also cause diffuse alopecia. It is important to evaluate thyroid function and to check for the presence of anemia with a complete blood count (CBC) in patients who present with diffuse, nonscarring alopecia.

Treatment: Telogen effluvium is a self-limited, reversible problem that usually resolves within 2 to 6 months. It may be prolonged if the underlying stress continues. For most patients, the stressful event will pass, and reassurance is all that is required. Regrowth is bound to occur.

There are no published studies on the efficacy of topical minoxidil for the treatment of telogen effluvium. However, minoxidil should be beneficial because it acts by shortening the resting phase of the hair cycle and converting more follicles into the growing phase.

Alopecia Areata

Clinical diagnosis: Alopecia areata is an idiopathic disorder characterized by well-circumscribed round or oval patches of complete hair loss with a clinically normal-appearing (ie, nonscarring) scalp. Alopecia areata most often affects the scalp and beard, but other areas, such as eyelashes and eyebrows, can also be affected. Characteristically short, blunt-tipped, and tapered at the base, 'exclamation point' hairs may be seen around the edges of bald spots.

Patients rarely lose all of their scalp hair (*alopecia totalis*) or all their body hair (*alopecia universalis*).

The prevalence of alopecia areata in the US general population is 1% to 2%. It affects both sexes equally, with onset occurring most often in early adulthood. From 20% to 25% of patients have a family history of the disorder. Alopecia areata is rarely associated with autoimmune diseases, such as Hashimoto's thyroiditis and pernicious anemia, and patients are otherwise generally healthy.

The pathogenesis of alopecia areata remains poorly understood, although an immunologic process is favored. A lymphocytic inflammatory infiltrate surrounds the affected hair bulbs and presumably has a role in the disease. In response to this autoimmune process, the hair matrices become arrested, but retain the capacity for normal hair regrowth after months or sometimes years. However, longstanding alopecia areata can lead to eventual fibrosis of the hair follicles.

Treatment: The treatment of alopecia areata depends on the extent of involvement and the patient's emotional need for hair regrowth. Because alopecia areata is considered to be immune-mediated rather than hormone-driven, intralesional steroids are typically prescribed. For localized disease, intralesional corticosteroid is often, at least temporarily, effective. Multiple superficial intralesional injections of triamcinolone acetonide (Kenalog-10®, Kenalog-40®) at a concentration of ≤10 mg/mL to the affected areas are given monthly. Regrowth is usually not noticed until after 4 to 8 weeks, and the monthly injections are usually continued for several more months. Superpotent topical steroids under occlusion are occasionally effective. Referral to a dermatologist for the treatment of alopecia areata is recommended, especially for cases that show no response to intralesional or topical steroids. Other treatment options used by dermatologists include systemic corticosteroids, topical anthralin, topical minoxidil, dinitrochlorobenzene (DNCB), and photochemotherapy with psoralen/ultraviolet light A (PUVA) using 8-methoxypsoralen (8-MOP®, Oxsoralen-Ultra®). Some patients with alopecia areata suffer emotional stress as a result of their hair loss and may benefit from psychological counseling.

Alopecia areata has a variable, unpredictable course. Most patients will have spontaneous recovery. However, relapses may occur. Duration of the condition for more than 1 year and extensive hair loss are poor prognostic signs.

Unwanted Facial Hair

Eflornithine hydrochloride cream, 13.9% (Vaniqa®) is the first topical prescription treatment for women with unwanted facial hair. In most cases, unwanted facial hair is caused by hereditary factors. However, some cases are caused by medical conditions, such as androgen excess disorder or polycystic ovary syndrome. Regardless of the cause, eflornithine appears to retard hair growth by interfering with the enzyme ornithine decarboxylase, which is found in the hair follicle needed for hair growth. This results in slower hair growth and improved appearance where eflornithine is applied.

Eflornithine is not a depilatory. Patients will likely need to continue using a hair removal method (eg, shaving, plucking) in conjunction with the drug's use.

Improvement in the condition occurs gradually and may not be seen until after 4 to 8 weeks of treatment. Improvement may take longer in some patients. The hair may return to the pretreatment condition when treatment with eflornithine is discontinued.

The most common side effects associated with eflornithine are minor skin irritations, such as temporary redness, hair bumps, stinging, burning, tingling, acne, or rash. In clinical trials, when side effects occurred, they were mild and generally resolved without medical treatment or discontinuation of eflornithine.

Appendix

Potency Rating of Commonly Used Topical Corticosteroids

Brand Name	Sizes	Generic Name
Group I		
Cordran® tape	24" and 80" rolls, 12 patches 2" x 3"	Flurandrenolide
Cormax® scalp application 0.05%	25 mL, 50 mL	Clobetasol propionate
Diprolene® ointment 0.05%	15 g, 50 g	Betamethasone dipropionate
Psorcon® ointment 0.05%	15 g, 30 g, 60 g	Diflorasone diacetate
Psorcon® E™ cream 0.05%	15 g, 30 g, 60 g	Diflorasone diacetate
Temovate® cream 0.05%	15 g, 30 g, 45 g, 60 g	Clobetasol propionate
Temovate® ointment 0.05%	15 g, 30 g, 45 g, 60 g	Clobetasol propionate
Temovate® scalp application 0.05%	25 mL, 50 mL	Clobetasol propionate
Ultravate® cream 0.05%	15 g, 50 g	Halobetasol propionate
Ultravate® ointment 0.05%	15 g, 50 g	Halobetasol propionate

Brand Name	Sizes	Generic Name
Group II		
ApexiCon® ointment 0.05%	30 g, 60 g	Diflorasone diacetate
ApexiCon® E cream 0.05%	30 g, 60 g	Diflorasone diacetate
Diprolene® AF cream 0.05%	15 g, 50 g	Betamethasone dipropionate
Elocon® ointment 0.1%	15 g, 45 g	Mometasone furoate
Halog® cream 0.1%	15 g, 30 g, 60 g, 240 g	Halcinonide
Lidex® cream 0.05%	15 g, 30 g, 60 g	Fluocinonide
Lidex® gel 0.05%	15 g, 30 g, 60 g	Fluocinonide
Lidex® ointment 0.05%	15 g, 30 g, 60 g	Fluocinonide
Topicort® cream 0.25%	15 g, 60 g	Desoximetasone
Topicort® ointment 0.25%	15 g, 60 g	Desoximetasone
Group III		
Cutivate® ointment 0.005%	15 g, 30 g, 60 g	Fluticasone propionate
Halog® ointment 0.1%	15 g, 30 g, 60 g, 240 g	Halcinonide
Lidex-E® cream 0.05%	15 g, 30 g, 60 g	Fluocinonide
Topicort® LP cream 0.05%	15 g, 60 g	Desoximetasone

Brand Name	Sizes	Generic Name
Group IV		
Elocon® cream 0.1%	15 g, 45 g	Mometasone furoate
Kenalog® ointment 0.1%	15 g, 60 g, 80 g	Triamcinolone acetonide
Synalar® ointment 0.025%	15 g, 60 g	Fluocinolone acetonide
Westcort® ointment 0.2%	15 g, 45 g, 60 g	Hydrocortisone valerate
Group V		
Cordran® cream 0.05%	15 g, 30 g, 60 g	Flurandrenolide
Cordran® lotion 0.05%	15 mL, 60 mL	Flurandrenolide
Cordran® ointment 0.05%	15 g, 30 g, 60 g	Flurandrenolide
Cutivate® cream 0.05%	15 g, 30 g, 60 g	Fluticasone propionate
Cutivate® lotion 0.05%	60 mL	Fluticasone propionate
Kenalog® cream 0.1%	15 g, 60 g, 80 g	Triamcinolone acetonide
Kenalog® lotion 0.1%	60 mL	Triamcinolone acetonide
Locoid® cream 0.1%	15 g, 45 g	Hydrocortisone butyrate
Synalar® cream 0.1%	15 g, 60 g	Fluocinolone acetonide
Westcort® cream 0.2%	15 g, 45 g, 60 g	Hydrocortisone valerate

Brand Name	Sizes	Generic Name
Group VI		
Aclovate® cream 0.05%	15 g, 45 g, 60 g	Alclometasone dipropionate
Aclovate® ointment 0.05%	15 g, 45 g, 60 g	Alclometasone dipropionate
DesOwen® cream 0.05%	15 g, 60 g, 90 g	Desonide
DesOwen® lotion 0.05%	60 mL, 120 mL	Desonide
DesOwen® ointment 0.05%	15 g, 60 g	Desonide
Synalar® solution 0.01%	20 mL, 60 mL	Fluocinolone acetonide
Synalar® cream 0.025%	15 g, 60 g	Fluocinolone acetonide

Group VII

Topicals with hydrocortisone, dexamethasone, flumethasone, prednisolone, and methylprednisolone

Index

A

viral shedding 74
vitamin A 26, 115
vitiligo 45, 46
vulvitis 63

W

warfarin (Coumadin®) 7, 10, 115
wart (condyloma cuminatum) 9, 10, 20, 41, 75, 76
  acuminate/venereal 78
  anogenital 78, 79
  common (verruca vulgaris) 75
  cutaneous nongenital 75, 77
  flat (verruca plana) 8, 75, 77
  genital 78
  mucosal 78
  plantar (verruca plantaris) 10, 75, 77
weeping 17, 72
wen 96

Westcort® 121
wheals 6, 12-14, 90, 93, 94
whiteheads 49
Wickham's striae 83
Wood's lamp 47
Wood's light examination 45
Wright's stain 15

X

xerosis 37

Y

yeast 14, 59, 60, 61, 63

Z

Ziana™ 49, 50
zinc 116
zinc pyrithione (Head & Shoulders®) 33, 62
Zostrix® 73
Zostrix®-HP 73
Zovirax® 42, 72

NOTES

Contemporary Guide to Dermatology™

Retail $19.95

Ordering Information

Prices (in U.S. dollars)

1 book:	$19.95 each
2-9 books:	$17.96 each
10-99 books:	$15.96 each
> 99 books:	Call 800-860-9544*

How to Order:

1. by telephone: 800-860-9544*
2. by fax: 215-860-9558
3. by Internet: www.HHCbooks.com
4. by mail: Handbooks in Health Care Co.
3 Terry Drive, Suite 201
Newtown, PA 18940

Shipping/Handling

**Books will be shipped via Priority Mail
or UPS Ground unless otherwise requested.**

1-3 books:	$6.00
4-9 books:	$8.00
10-14 books:	$11.00
15-24 books:	$13.00
> 24 books:	Plus shipping
International orders:	Please inquire

*Please call between 9 AM and 5 PM EST Monday through Friday, 800-860-9544.

Pennsylvania residents must add 6% sales tax.

Prices good through March 31, 2008